MEDICAL ABBREVIATIONS:

4200 Conveniences at the Expense of Communications and Safety

Third Edition

Neil M. Davis, M.S., Pharm.D.
Professor of Pharmacy, Temple University
School of Pharmacy, Philadelphia, PA,
Editor-in-Chief, Hospital Pharmacy

published by

Neil M. Davis Associates
1143 Wright Drive
Huntingdon Valley, PA 19006
(215)-947-1862 (or 1752)

i

Library of Congress Catalog Card Number: 86-71890

Copyright © 1987, 1985, and 1983 by Neil M. Davis Associates

First edition, 1983, titled, "1700 Medical Abbreviations:
Convenience at the Expense of Communications and Safety"

Second edition, 1985, titled, "Medical Abbreviations:
2300 Conveniences at the Expense of Communications
and Safety

ISBN 0-931431-03-4

The user must exercise care in that the meaning shown in
this book may not be the one intended by a writer. When
there is doubt, the writer must be contacted for clarification.

Preface

L isted are 4200 current abbreviations, acronyms and symbols and 5800 of their possible meanings. This list has been compiled to assist individuals in reading medical records and prescriptions. The list only scratches the surface of abbreviations in use and their many possible meanings as new ones are being coined every day.

The fact that some abbreviations are in capital letters while others are in lower case, some have slashes, and periods may or may not be used, is not critical to their meaning since there is individual variation in the way abbreviations are written.

Abbreviations are a convenience, a time saver, a space saver and a way of avoiding the possibility of misspelling words. A price is paid for their use. Abbreviations are sometimes not understood or are interpreted incorrectly. Their use lengthens the time needed to train individuals in the health fields, at times delays the care of patients and occasionally results in their being harmed.

The publication of this list of abbreviations is not an endorsement of their legitimacy, a guarantee that the intended meaning has been correctly captured, or an indication that they are in common use. Where uncertainty exists, the writer must be contacted for clarification.

Hospitals are wisely required by the Joint Commission on Accreditation of Hospitals to formulate an approved list of abbreviations. Every attempt should be made to restrict this list to common abbreviations that are understood by all health professionals who must work with medical records. There are certain dangerous abbreviations that should not be approved, and a warning should be issued about their use (See Table 1 as well as notes in the text).

Many inherent problems associated with abbreviations contribute to or cause errors. Reports of such errors have been published routinely.[1-3]

Table 1. Some dangerous abbreviations

Problem term	Reason	Suggested term
O.D. for once daily	Interpreted as right eye	Write "once daily"
q.o.d. for every other day	Interpreted as meaning once daily or read as q.i.d.	Write "every other day"
q.d. for once daily	Read or interpreted as q.i.d.	Write "once daily"
q.n. for every night	Read as every hour	Write "every night," "H.S." or nightly
q hs for every night	Read as every hour	Use "HS" or "at bedtime"
U for Unit	Read as 0, 4, 6 or cc.	Write "unit"
O.J. for orange juice	Read as OD or OS	Write "orange juice"
µg (microgram)	When handwritten, misread as mg	Write "mcg"
sq or sub q for subcutaneous	The q is read as every	Use "subcut"
Chemical symbols	Not understood or misunderstood	Write full name
Lettered abbreviations for drug names	Not understood or misunderstood	Use generic or trade name
Apothecary symbols or terms	Not understood or misunderstood	Use metric system
per os or by mouth	OS read as left eye	Use "by mouth," "orally," or "P.O."
D/C for discharge	Interpreted as discontinue (orders for discharge medications result in premature discontinuance of current medication)	Write "discharge"
T/d	Read as T.I.D.	Use "once daily"

Abbreviations can be confused by the prescriber. For example, a physician prescribed "5 FU" when he wanted to prescribe flucytosine. 5 FU is fluorouracil, while flucytosine is 5 FC. The reverse has also been reported. Another physician incorrectly prescribed "5 FU" when he thought he was ordering floxuridine (FUDR).

Abbreviations can easily be misread or interpreted in a manner not intended. For example:

(1) "HCT250 mg" was intended to mean hydrocortisone 250 mg but was interpreted as hydrochlorothiazide 50 mg (HCTZ50 mg).

(2) A physician prescribed MTX. The order was interpreted as mustargen rather than methotrexate. MTX was confused with HN_2.

(3) The handwritten U for unit has been mistaken for a zero, causing a tenfold error. The handwritten U has also been read as the number four and as cc. The abbreviation "U" for unit is the most dangerous one in the book, having caused numerous 10 fold insulin overdoses. The word unit should never be abbreviated.

(4) OD meant to signify once daily has caused Lugol's solution to be given in the right eye.

(5) OJ, meant to signify orange juice, looked like OS and caused Saturated Solution of Potassium Iodide to be given in the left eye.

(6) Na Warfarin (Sodium Warfarin) was read as "No Warfarin."

(7) The abbreviation "s̄" for without has been thought to mean "with" (c̄).

(8) The order for PT, intended to signify a laboratory test order for prothrombin time, resulted in the ordering of a physical therapy consultation.

(9) The abbreviation, "TAB", meant to signify Triple Antibiotic, (a coined name for a hospital sterile antibiotic mixture), caused a patient to have their wound irrigated with a diet soda.

Many abbreviations have several meanings.

CF = cystic fibrosis; Caucasian female; calcium leucovorin (citrovorum factor); complement fixation; cancer-free; cardiac failure; coronary flow; contractile force; cephalothin; Christmas factor; count fingers

CPM = cyclophosphamide; chlorpheniramine maleate, continuous passive motion; continue present management; central pontine myelinolysis; counts per minute

PBZ = phenylbutazone; pyribenzamine; phenoxybenzamine

CPZ = chlorpromazine; Compazine®

DW = dextrose in water; distilled water; deionized water

MS = morphine sulfate; multiple sclerosis; mitral stenosis; musculoskeletal; medical student; minimal support; muscle strength; mental status

NBM = no bowel movement; normal bowel movement; nothing by mouth

One must wonder how often abbreviations are just skipped over by the reader of a medical record because the meaning is unknown or ambiguous. How many millions of health professional manhours are spent each year asking other health professionals what the meaning of an obscure abbreviation is? How many times is therapy or a diagnostic test delayed because an abbreviation is not understood? How much more difficult is it to train health professionals so they can understand the abbreviations used?

An examination of the following list is a testimonial to the problems and dangers associated with most undefined abbreviations.

The assistance of Aphirudee Poshakrishma, former teaching assistant, Temple University School of Pharmacy, Philadelphia, PA; Michael R. Cohen, Director of Pharmacy Service, Quakertown Community Hospital, Quakertown, PA; Ann Sandt Kishbaugh, J.B. Lippincott, Philadelphia and all the others that helped is gratefully acknowledged.

References

1. Davis NM, Cohen MR. Medication errors: causes and prevention. Philadelphia: Geo. F. Stickley & Co., 1981.

2. Cohen MR. Medication error reports. Hosp Pharm (appears monthly from 1975 to the present).

3. Cohen MR. Medication errors. Nursing 87 (appears monthly, starting in Nursing 77, to the present).

4. Adapted from Bates B. A guide to physical examinations. 3rd ed. Philadelphia: J.B. Lippincott, 1983.

Please forward any additional meanings for these abbreviations, additional abbreviations and their meanings, or corrections to the author so that the list can be updated. Thank you. Dr. Neil M. Davis, 1143 Wright Drive, Huntingdon Valley, PA 19006.

A

A — assessment; artery; ambulatory; apical; alive

A$_2$ — aortic second sound

AA — Alcoholic Anonymous; amino acid; achievement age; authorized absence; auto accident; active assistive; arm ankle (pulse ratio)

AAA — abdominal aortic aneurysmectomy (aneurysm)

AAC — antimicrobial agent-associated colitis

AAL — anterior axillary line

AAN — analgesic-associated nephropathy; attending's admission notes; analgesic abuse nephropathy

AAO × 3 — awake and oriented to time, place and person

AAP — assessment adjustment pass

AAPC — antibiotic acquired pseudomembranous colitis

AAROM — active assistive range of motion

AAS — atlantoaxis subluxation

AAV — adeno-associated virus

AAVV — accumulated alveolar ventilatory volume

Ab — abortion; antibody

A & B — apnea and bradycardia

ABC — artificial beta cells; absolute band counts

ABCDE — botulism toxoid pentavalent

Abd — abdomen; abdominal

ABDCT — atrial bolus dynamic computer tomography

ABDIC — a drug combination protocol

ABDV — a drug combination protocol

ABE — acute bacterial endocarditis; botulism equine trivalent antitoxin

ABG — arterial blood gases

ABI — atherothrombotic brain infarction

ABL — allograft bound lymphocytes

ABLB — alternate binaural loudness balance

ABMT — autologous bone marrow transplantation

ABN — abnormality(ies)

A.B.N.M. — American Board of Nuclear Medicine

abnor. — abnormal

ABR — absolute bed rest; auditory brain (evoked) responses

ABS — at bedside; admitting blood sugar; absorption; absorbed

ABT — aminopyrine breath test

ABVD — adriamycin, bleomycin, vinblastine and dacarbazine (DTIC)

ABW — actual body weight

ABx — antibiotics

AC	acute; before meals; antecubital; acetate; acromio-clavicular; abdominal circumference; anchored catheter; air conduction; assist control; air conditioned	ACPP PF	acid phosphatase prostatic fluid
		ACS	American Cancer Society
A/C	anterior chamber of the eye	ACSW	Academy of Certified Social Workers
5-AC	azacitidine	ACT	activated clotting time; allergen challenge test
ACA	acyclovir; anterior cerebral artery	ACT-D	dactinomycin
ACB	antibody-coated bacteria	Act Ex	active exercise
		ACTH	corticotropin (adrenocorticotrophic hormone)
AC & BC	air and bone conduction		
ACBE	air contrast barium enema	ACTSEB	anterior chamber tube shunt encircling band
ACC	accommodation; administrative control center; adenoid cystic carcinomas	ACV	atrial/carotid/ventricular; acyclovir
		AD	accident dispensary; right ear; Alzheimer's disease
ACD	acid-citrate-dextrose; anterior chest diameter; absolute cardiac dullness; dactinomycin; anterior chamber diameter	ADA	American Diabetes Association; adenosine deaminase
		ADAU	adolescent drug abuse unit
		ADCC	antibody-dependent cellular cytotoxicity
ACE	angiotensin-converting enzyme	ADC	Aid to Dependent Children
ACH	adrenal cortical hormone	ADD	attention deficit disorder; adduction
ACh	acetylcholine	ADDU	alcohol and drug dependence unit
ACI	aftercare instructions		
ACL	anterior cruciate ligament	ADEM	acute disseminating encephalomyelitis
ACLS	advanced cardiac life support	ADH	antidiuretic hormone
		ADL	activities of daily living
ACP	acid phosphatase	ad lib	as desired; at liberty
AC-PH	acid phosphatase	ADM	admission; doxorubicin

Ad-OAP	doxorubicin/vincristine/cytarabine/prednisone	A/G	albumin to globulin ratio
adol	adolescent	Ag	antigen
ADR	adverse drug reaction; doxorubicin (Adriamycin®); acute dystonic reaction	AG	anti-gravity; aminoglycoside; anion gap
		AGA	appropriate for gestational age; acute gonococcal arthritis
ADRIA	doxorubicin (Adriamycin®)	AGD	agar gel diffusion
ADS	anonymous donor's sperm; anatomical dead space	AGE	angle of greatest extension
		AGF	angle of greatest flexion
ADT	anticipate discharge tomorrow	AGG	agammaglobulinemia
		aggl.	agglutination
AE	above elbow (amputation); air entry	AGL	acute granulocytic leukemia
AEC	at earliest convenience	AGN	acute glomerulonephritis
AED	automated external defibrillator	Ag NO₃	silver nitrate
AEG	air encephalogram	AGPT	agar-gel precipitation test
AER	acoustic evoked response; auditory evoked response	AGS	adrenogenital syndrome
		AH	antihyaluronidase
Aer. M.	aerosol mask	AHA	autoimmune hemolytic anemia; acetohydroxamic acid
Aer. T.	aerosol tent		
AES	anti-embolic stockings		
AF	atrial fibrillation; acid-fast; anterior fontanel; amniotic fluid	AHC	acute hemorrhagic conjunctivitis; acute hemorrhagic cystitis
		AHD	autoimmune hemolytic disease
AFB	acid-fast bacilli; aorto-femoral bypass	AHF	antihemophilic factor
AFC	air filled cushions	AHFS	American Hospital Formulary Service
AFDC	Aid to Family and Dependent Children	AHG	antihemophilic globulin
A. fib.	atrial fibrillation		
AFO	ankle-foot orthosis	AHM	ambulatory Holter monitoring
AFP	alpha-fetoprotein		
AFV	amniotic fluid volume	AHT	autoantibodies to human thyroglobulin
AFVSS	afebrile, vital signs stable		

AI	aortic insufficiency; artificial insemination; allergy index	A/K, AK	above knee (amputation)
A & I	Allergy and Immunology (department)	AKA	above-knee amputation; also known as; alcoholic ketoacidosis; all known allergies
AI-Ab	anti-insulin antibody	ALA	aminolevulinic acid
AICA	anterior inferior communicating artery; anterior inferior cerebellar artery	ALAT	alanine transaminase (alanine aminotransferase; SGPT)
AICD	automatic implantable cardioverter/defibrillator	Alb	albumin
		ALC	acute lethal catatonia; alcohol
AID	artificial insemination donor; automatic implantable defibrillator	ALC R	alcohol rub
		ALD	alcohol liver disease; aldolase; adrenoleukodystrophy
AIDS	acquired immune deficiency syndrome	ALDOST	aldosterone
AIE	acute inclusion body encephalitis	ALFT	abnormal liver function tests
AIF	aortic-iliac-femoral	ALG	antilymphocyte globulin
AIH	artificial insemination with husband's sperm	alk	alkaline
AIHA	autoimmune hemolytic anemia	ALK-P	alkaline phosphatase
AILD	angioimmunoblastic lymphadenopathy (with dysproteinemia)	ALL	acute lymphocytic leukemia; allergy
		ALM	acral lentiginous melanoma
AIMS	abnormal involuntary movement scale	ALMI	anterolateral myocardial infarction
AINS	anti-inflammatory non-steroidal	Al(OH)$_3$	aluminum hydroxide
AION	anterior ischemic optic neuropathy	ALS	amyotrophic lateral sclerosis; acute lateral sclerosis; advanced life support
AIP	acute intermittent porphyria		
AIR	accelerate idioventricular rhythm	ALT	alanine transaminase (SGPT); Argon laser trabeculoplasty
AIVR	accelerated idioventricular rhythm		
AJ	ankle jerk	ALWMI	anterolateral wall myocardial infarct

AM	morning; myopic astigmatism; amalgam	AMSIT	portion of the mental status examination: A—appearance, M—mood, S—sensorium, I—intelligence, T—thought process
AMA	against medical advice; antimitochondrial antibody; American Medical Association		
		amt.	amount
AMAP	as much as possible	AMY	amylase
A-MAT	amorphous material	ANA	antinuclear antibody
Amb	ambulate; ambulatory	ANAD	anorexia nervosa and associated disorders
AMC	arm muscle circumference	ANC	absolute neutrophil count
AMD	age-related macular degeneration	AND	anterior nasal discharge
AMegL	acute megokaryo-blastic leukemia	ANDA	Abbreviated New Drug Application
AMG	acoustic myography	anes	anesthesia
AMI	acute myocardial infarction; ami-triptyline	ANF	antinuclear factor; atrial natriuretic factor
AML	acute myelogenous leukemia	ANG	angiogram
		ANLL	acute nonlymphoblastic leukemia
AMM	agnogenic myeloid metaplasia	ANOVA	analysis of variance
AMMOL	acute myelomono-blastic leukemia	ANS	autonomic nervous system; answer
amnio	amniocentesis	ant.	anterior
AMOL	acute monoblastic leukemia	ante	before
		A & O	alert and oriented
AMP	amputation; ampul; ampicillin; adenosine monophosphate	AOAP	as often as possible
		AOB	alcohol on breath
		ao-il	aorta-iliac
A-M pr	Austin-Moore prosthesis	AOC	area of concern
		AODM	adult onset diabetes mellitus
AMR	alternating motor rates	AOM	acute otitis media
AMS	amylase; acute moun-tain sickness	AOP	aortic pressure
		A&O × 3	awake and oriented to person, place and time
AMV	assisted mechanical ventilation	A&O × 4	awake and oriented to person, place time and date
m-AMSA	acridinyl anisidide		

11

AOSD	adult-onset Still's disease	APTT	activated partial thromboplastin time
A&P	anterior and posterior; auscultation and percussion; assessment and plans	aq	water
		aq dest	distilled water
		AR	aortic regurgitation
AP	anterior-posterior (x-ray); antepartum; apical pulse; appendicitis	A&R	advised and released
		A-R	apical-radial (pulse)
		ARA-A	vidarabine
		ARA-C	cytarabine
$A_2 > P_2$	second aortic sound greater than second pulmonic sound	ARB	any reliable brand
		ARC	anomalous retinal correspondence; American Red Cross; AIDS related complex
APAP	acetaminophen		
APB	atrial premature beat; abductor pollicis brevis	ARD	adult respiratory distress; acute respiratory disease; antibiotic removal device
APC	aspirin, phenacetin and caffeine; atrial premature contraction		
		ARDS	adult respiratory distress syndrome
APCD	adult polycystic disease		
APD	automated peritoneal dialysis; atrial premature depolarization	ARF	acute renal failure; acute rheumatic fever; acute respiratory failure
APE	acute psychotic episode	ARLD	alcohol related liver disease
APKD	adult polycystic kidney disease		
		ARM	artificial rupture of membranes
APL	acute promyelocytic leukemia; abductor pollicis longus; accelerated painless labor; chorionic gonadotropin		
		AROM	active range of motion; artifical rupture of membranes
		arr	arrive
APO	a drug combination protocol	ARS	antirabies serum
		A.R.R.T.	American Registry of Radiologic Technologists
apo E	apolipoprotein E		
APPG	aqueous procaine penicillin G (dangerous terminology; for intramuscular use only)		
		ART	automated reagin test (for syphilis); arterial
		ARV	AIDS related virus
appr.	approximate	AS	aortic stenosis; activated sleep; anal sphincter; left ear; ankylosing spondylitis
appt.	appointment		
APR	abdominoperineal resection		

ASA	acetylsalicyclic acid (aspirin); arginino-succinate; American Society of Anesthesiologists		ASCVD	arteriosclerotic cardio-vascular disease
			ASD	atrial septal defect
			ASE	acute stress erosion
			ASH	asymmetric septal hypertrophy
ASA I	Healthy patient with localized pathological process		ASHD	arteriosclerotic heart disease
ASA II	A patient with mild to moderate systemic disease		ASIS	anterior superior iliac spine
			ASK	antistreptokinase
ASA III	A patient with severe systemic disease limiting activity but not incapacitating		ASL	antistreptolysin (titer)
			ASLO	antistreptolysin-O
			AsM	myopic astigmatism
			ASMI	anteroseptal myocardial infarction
ASA IV	A patient with incapacitating systemic disease		ASO	antistreptolysin-O titer; arteriosclerosis obliterans
ASA V	Moribund patient not expected to live.		ASOT	antistreptolysin-O titer
			ASP	acute suppurative parotitis
	(These are American Society of Anesthesiologists' patient classifications. Emergency operations are designated by "E" after the classification).		ASS	anterior superior supine
			AST	aspartate transaminase (SGOT); astigmatism; astemizole
			ASTZ	antistreptozyme test
			ASU	acute stroke unit
			ASVD	arteriosclerotic vessel disease
ASAA	acquired severe aplastic anemia		AT	applanation tonometry; atraumatic; anti-thrombin
ASAP	as soon as possible		ATB	antibiotic
ASAT	aspartate transaminase (aspartate amino-transferase) (SGOT)		ATC	around the clock
			ATD	antithyroid drug(s); autoimmune thyroid disease
ASB	anesthesia standby; asymptomatic bacteriuria		At Fib	atrial fibrillation
			ATG	antithymocyte globulin
ASC	ambulatory surgery center; altered state of consciousness		ATHR	angina threshold heart rate

ATL	Achilles tendon lengthening; atypical lymphocytes; adult T-cell leukemia	AVR	aortic valve replacement
ATLS	advanced trauma life support	AVS	atriovenous shunt
ATN	acute tubular necrosis	AVSS	afebrile, vital signs stable
ATNC	atraumatic normocephalic	AVT	atypical ventricular tachycardia
aTNM	autopsy staging of cancer	A&W	alive and well
		A waves	atrial contraction waves
ATNR	asymmetrical tonic neck reflux	AWI	anterior wall infarct
ATP	adenosine triphosphate	AWOL	absent without leave
ATPase	adenosine triphosphatase	ax	axillary
		AZA	azathioprine
ATPS	ambient temperature & pressure, saturated with water vapor	5 AZA	azacitidine
		AZQ	diaziquone
		AZT	azidothymidine
ATR	atrial; Achilles tendon reflex	A-Z test	Ascheim-Zondek test; diagnostic test for pregnancy
ATT	arginine tolerance test		
AT 10	dihydrotachysterol		
AU	both ears; gold; allergenic units		

B

AUC	area under the curve	B	bacillus; bands; bloody; black; both; buccal
AV	arteriovenous; atrioventricular; auditory-visual		
		B_1	thiamine HCl
		B_2	riboflavin
AVA	arteriovenous anastomosis	B_6	pyridoxine HCl
		B_7	biotin
AVD	apparent volume of distribution	B_8	adenosine phosphate
		B_{12}	cyanocobalamin
AVF	arteriovenous fistula	Ba	barium
AVH	acute viral hepatitis	BA	blood alcohol; Bourns assist; backache; bile acid
AVM	atriovenous malformation		
AVN	atrioventricular node; arteriovenous nicking; avascular necrosis	BAC	blood alcohol concentration; benzalkonium chloride; buccoaxiocervical
AVP	arginine vasopressin		

BACOP	bleomycin, adriamycin, cyclophosphamide, vincristine, prednisone	BCAA	branched-chain amino acids
BAD	dipolar affective disorder	BCC	basal cell carcinoma
		BCD	basal cell dysplasia
BaE	barium enema	BCE	basal cell epithelioma
BAE	bronchial artery embolization	B cell	large lymphocyte
		BCG	bacillus Calmette-Guerin vaccine
BAEP	brain stem auditory evoked potential	BCL	basic cycle length
BAERs	brain stem auditory evoked responses	BCNU	carmustine
		BCP	birth control pills
BAL	British antilewisite (dimercaprol); blood alcohol level; bronchoalveolar lavage	BCS	battered child syndrome; Budd-Chiari syndrome
		BD	bronchial drainage; birth defect; brain dead
BAO	basal acid output		
BAP	blood agar plate	BDAE	Boston Diagnostic Aphasia Examination
baso.	basophil		
BAVP	balloon aortic valvuloplasty	BDI SF	Beck's Depression Index-Short Form
BB	blow bottle; bed bath; buffer base; bowel or bladder; breakthrough bleeding; blood bank	BDP	beclomethasone diproprionate
		BDR	background diabetic retinopathy
BBA	born before arrival	BE	barium enema; below elbow; bread equivalent; bacterial endocarditis; base excess
BBB	bundle branch block; blood-brain barrier		
BBBB	bilateral bundle branch block		
BBD	benign breast disease	BEC	bacterial endocarditis
BBM	banked breast milk	BEE	basal energy expenditure
BBS	bilateral breath sounds		
BBT	basal body temperature	BEI	butanol-extractable iodine
BC	bone conduction; blood culture; birth control; Bourn control; bed and chair	BEP	brain stem evoked potentials
		BF	black female
		BFP	biologic false positive
BCA	balloon catheter angioplasty; basal cell atypia; brachiocephalic artery	BFT	bentonite flocculation test
		BFU_e	erythroid burst-forming unit

BG	blood glucose	Bkg	background
BGC	basal-ganglion calcification	BLB	Boothby-Lovelace-Bulbulian (oxygen mask)
BHC	benzene hexachloride		
BHI	biosynthetic human insulin	bl cult	blood culture
		BLE	both lower extremities
BHN	bridging hepatic necrosis	BLESS	bath, laxative, enema, shampoo & shower
BHS	beta-hemolytic strepto-cocci	BLEO	bleomycin sulfate
		BLM	bleomycin sulfate
BI	bowel impaction	BLOBS	bladder obstruction
BIB	brought in by	BLS	basic life support
BID	twice daily	B.L. unit	Bessey-Lowry units
BIG 6	analysis of 6 serum components	BM	bowel movement; bone marrow; black male; breast milk
BIH	benign intracranial hypertension; bilateral inguinal hernia		
		BMA	bone marrow aspirate
		BMC	bone marrow cells
bil.	bilateral	BMI	body mass index
BILAT SLC	bilateral short leg case	BMJ	bones, muscles, joints
		BMR	basal metabolic rate
BILAT SXO	bilateral salpingo-oophorectomy	BMT	bone marrow trans-plant; bilateral myrin-gotomy tubes
Bili	bilirubin		
BILI-C	conjugated bilirubin	BMTU	bone marrow trans-plant unit
BIMA	bilateral internal mammary arteries		
		BNO	bladder neck obstruction
BiPD	biparietal diameter		
bisp	bispinous diameter	BNR	bladder neck retraction
B.I.W.	twice a week (this is a dangerous abbrevi-ation)	BO	behavior objective; body odor; bowel ob-struction
BJ	bone and joint	B & O	belladonna & opium
BJE	bones, joints, and examination	BOA	born on arrival; born out of asepsis
BJM	bones, joints, and muscles	BOB	ball on back
		BOLD	bleomycin, vincristine, (Oncovin) lomustine and dacarbazine
BJ protein	Bence-Jones protein		
BK	below knee (ampu-tation)		
		BOM	bilateral otitis media
BKA	below knee amputation	BOO	bladder outlet obstruction
bkft	breakfast		

BOT	base of tongue	BS	blood sugar; breath sounds; bowel sounds; before sleep
B.O.W.	bag of water		
BP	blood pressure; benzoyl peroxide; British Pharmacopeia; bed pan	B & S	Bartholin & Skene (glands)
BPD	biparietal diameter; bronchopulmonary dysplasia	BSA	body surface area
		BSB	body surface burned
BPF	bronchopleural fistula	BSC	bedside commode
BPH	benign prostatic hypertrophy	BSE	breast self-examination
		BSER	brain stem evoked responses
BPG	bypass graft	BSF	busulfan
BPL	benzylpenicilloyl-polylysine	BSGA	beta Streptococcus group A
BPM	breaths per minute; beats per minute	BSO	bilateral salpingo-oophorectomy
BPN	bacitracin, polymyxin B, and neomycin sulfate	BSOM	bilateral serous otitis media
		BSP	bromsulphalein
BPRS	Brief Psychiatric Rate Scale	BSPM	body surface potential mapping
BPSD	bronchopulmonary segmental drainage	BSS®	balanced salt solution; black silk sutures
BPV	benign paroxysmal vertigo	BSSG	sitogluside
Bq	becquerel	BSU	Bartholin, Skene's, urethra
BR	bedrest; bridge; Benzing retrograde; bathroom	BSW	Bachelor of Social Work
BRA	brain	BT	breast tumor; brain tumor; bedtime; bituberous; bladder tumor; blood transfusion
BRAO	branch retinal artery occlusion		
BRATT	bananas, rice, apple-sauce, tea, & toast	BTB	break-through bleeding
BRB	blood-retinal barrier	BTFS	breast tumor frozen section
BRBPR	bright red blood per rectum	BTL	bilateral tubal ligation
BRJ	brachial radialis jerk	BTPS	body temperature pressure saturated
BRM	biological response modifiers	BTR	bladder tumor recheck
		BUdR	bromodeoxyurdine
BRP	bathroom privileges	BUE	both upper extremities

BUN	blood urea nitrogen; bunion
BUR	back-up rate (ventilator)
BUS	Bartholin, urethral and Skene's glands
BVL	bilateral vas ligation
BW	body weight; birth weight; body water
B & W	Black and White (milk of magnesia & aromatic cascara fluid extract)
BWCS	bagged white cell study
BWFI	bacteriostatic water for injection
BWS	battered woman syndrome
ΦBZ	phenylbutazone
Bx	biopsy
BX BS	Blue Cross and Blue Shield
BZDZ	benzodiazepine

C

C	clubbing; cyanosis; carbohydrate; centigrade; ascorbic acid; Celsius; hundred; Catholic
$\overline{c}$	with
C_1	first cervical vertebra
C_1 to C_9	precursor molecules of the complement system
CII	controlled substance, class 2
CA	carcinoma; chronologic age; cardiac arrest; coronary artery; carotid artery

C&A	Clinitest and Acetest
CAA	crystalline amino acids
CAB	coronary artery bypass
CABG	coronary artery bypass graft
CaBI	calcium bone index
CABS	coronary artery bypass surgery
CACI	computer assisted continuous infusion
CACP	cisplatin
CAD	coronary artery disease
CAE	cellulose acetate electrophoresis
CAF	cyclophosphamide, doxorubicin and fluorouracil
CAFT	Clinitron air fluidized therapy
CAH	chronic active hepatitis; chronic aggressive hepatitis; congenital adrenal hyperplasia
CAL	calories; callus; chronic airflow limitation
CALD	chronic active liver disease
CALGB	Cancer and Leukemia Group B
CALLA	common acute lymphoblastic leukemia antigen
CAMF	cyclophosphamide, adriamycin, methotrexate and fluorouracil
CAMP	cyclophosphamide, doxorubicin, methotrexate and procarbazine
CAN	cord around neck
CAO	chronic airway (airflow) obstruction

CAP	capsule; cyclophosphamide; doxorubicin and cisplatin; compound action potentials	CBI	continuous bladder irrigation
		CBN	chronic benign neutropenia
CAPD	chronic ambulatory peritoneal dialysis	CBR	complete bedrest; chronic bedrest; carotid bodies resected
CAR	cardiac ambulation routine	CBS	chronic brain syndrome
CARB	carbohydrate	CBZ	carbamazepine
CAS	carotid artery stenosis	CC	chief complaint; chronic complainer; clean catch (urine); cubic centimeter (mL); critical condition; cord compression; creatinine clearance; cerebral concussion
CAT	computed axial tomography; children's apperception test; cataract		
cath.	catheter; catheterization		
CAV	cyclophosphamide, doxorubicin and vincristine		
		CCA	common carotid artery
CAVB	complete atrioventricular block	CCAP	capsule cartilage articular preservation
CAVC	common arterioventricular canal	CCB	calcium channel blocker(s)
CAVH	continuous ateriovenous hemofiltration	CC & C	colony count and culture
CB	code blue; chronic bronchitis; cesarean birth; chair and bed	CCE	clubbing, cyanosis, and edema
		CCF	crystal-induced chemotactic factor; compound comminuted fracture
C & B	crown and bridge		
CBA	chronic bronchitis and asthma		
		CCFE	cyclophosphamide, cisplatin, fluorouracil and estramustine
CBC	complete blood count; carbenicillin		
CBD	common bile duct; closed bladder drainage	CCHD	cyanotic congenital heart disease
CBF	cerebral blood blow	CCI	chronic coronary insufficiency
CBFS	cerebral blood flow studies	CCK	cholecystokinin
CBFV	cerebral blood flow velocity	CCK-OP	cholecystokinin octapeptide
CBG	capillary blood glucose	CCK-PZ	cholecystokinin-pancreozymin

CCM	cyclophosphamide, lomustine and methotrexate
CCMSU	clean catch midstream urine
CCNU	lomustine
C-collar	cervical collar
CCPD	continuous cycling (cyclical) peritoneal dialysis
CCR	continuous complete remission
CCRU	critical care recovery unit
CCT	congenitally corrected transposition (of the great vessels)
CCTGA	congenitally corrected transposition of the great arteries
CCT in PET	crude coal tar in petroleum
CCTV	closed circuit television
CCU	coronary care unit
CCUP	colpocystourethropexy
CCX	complications
CD	Crohn's Disease; continuous drainage; cesarean delivery
C/D	cup to disc ratio
C&D	curettage and desiccation; cytoscopy and dilatation
CDA	chenodeoxycholic acid (chenodiol); congenital dyserythropoietic anemia
CDAI	Crohn's Disease Activity Index
CDB	cough, deep breath

CDC	Centers for Disease Control; chenodeoxycholic acid; Cancer Detection Center; calculated day of confinement
CDCA	chenodeoxycholic acid (chenodiol)
CDDP	cisplatin
CDE	common duct exploration
CDH	congenital dysplasia of the hip; chronic daily headache
CDLE	chronic discoid lupus erythematosus
cdyn	dynamic compliance
CE	central episiotomy; continuing education; cardiac enlargement; contrast echocardiology
CEA	carcinoembryonic antigen; carotid endarterectomy
CECT	contrast enhancement computed tomography
CEI	continuous extravascular infusion
CEO	chief executive officer
CEP	congenital erythropoietic porphyria; countercurrent electrophoresis
CEPH	cephalic; cephalosporin
CEPH FLOC	cephalin flocculation
CE&R	central episiotomy & repair
CERA	cortical evoked response audiometry

CERV	cervical	CH	child; chronic; chest; chief; crown-heal; convalescent hospital; cluster headache
CES	cognitive environmental stimulation		
CF	cystic fibrosis; Caucasian female; calcium leucovorin (citrovorum factor); complement fixation; cardiac failure; cancer-free; count fingers; Christmas factor; cephalothin; contractile force	c̄ hold	withhold
		CHAD	cyclophosphamide, adriamycin, cisplatin and hexamethylmelamine
		CHAI	continuous hepatic artery infusion
		CHB	complete heart block
		CH₃– CCNU	semustine
CFA	common femoral artery; complete Freund's adjuvant	CHD	congenital heart disease; childhood diseases
CFM	close fitting mask	CHF	congestive heart failure; Crimean hemorrhagic fever
CFP	cystic fibrosis protein		
CFS	cancer family syndrome	CHFV	combined high frequency of ventilation
CFT	complement fixation test		
CF test	complement fixation test	CHG	change
		CHI	closed head injury
CFU	colony forming units	CHO	carbohydrate
CFU-S	colony forming unit—spleen	chol	cholesterol
		CHOP	cyclophosphamide/doxorubicin/vincristine/prednisone
CG	cholecystogram		
CGB	chronic gastrointestinal (tract) bleeding	chr.	chronic
		CHRS	congenital hereditary retinoschisis
CGD	chronic granulomatous disease		
		CHS	Chediak-Higashi syndrome
CGI	Clinical Global Impression (scale)		
		CHU	closed head unit
CGL	chronic granulocytic leukemia; with correction/with glasses	CI	cesium implant; complete iridectomy; cardiac index
CGN	chronic glomerulonephritis	Ci	curie(s)
		CIA	chronic idiopathic anhidrosis
CGTT	cortisol glucose tolerance test		

CIAED	collagen induced autoimmune ear disease
CIB	cytomegalic inclusion bodies; Carnation Instant Breakfast
CIBD	chronic inflammatory bowel disease
CIC	circulating immune complexes
CICE	combined intracapsular cataract extraction
CICU	cardiac intensive care unit
CID	cytomegalic inclusion disease
CIDP	chronic inflammatory demyelinating polyradineuropathy
CIDS	continuous insulin delivery system; cellular immunodeficiency syndrome
CIE	counterimmunoelectrophoresis; crossed immunoelectrophoresis
CIN	chronic interstitial nephritis; cervical intraepithelial neoplasia
Circ	circumcision; circumference
CIS	carcinoma in situ
CISCA	cisplatin, Cytoxan® & Adriamycin®
Cis-DDP	cisplatin
CIU	chronic idiopathic urticaria
CJD	Creutzfeldt-Jakob Disease
CK	check; creatine kinase
CK-MB	a creatine kinase isoenzyme
cl.	cloudy

Cl	chloride
CL	critical list
CLA	community living arrangements
Clav	clavicle
CLB	chlorambucil
CLBBB	complete left bundle branch block
CLC	cork leather and celastic (orthotic)
CLD	chronic lung disease; chronic liver disease
CLF	cholesterol-lecithin flocculation
CLH	chronic lobular hepatitis
CLL	chronic lymphocytic leukemia
CLLE	columnar-lined lower esophagus
cl liq	clear liquid
CLO	cod liver oil; close
CL & P	cleft lip & palate
CLT	chronic lymphocytic thyroiditis
CL VOID	clean voided specimen
clysis	hypodermoclysis
cm	centimeter
CM	costal margin; capreomycin; continuous murmur; Caucasian male; centimeter; contrast media; cochlear microphonics; culture media; common migraine
CMBBT	cervical mucous basal body temperature
CMC	chloramphenicol; carboxymethylcellulose; chronic mucocutaneous moniliasis

CME	cystoid macular edema; continuing medical education
CMF	cyclophosphamide/methotrexate; fluorouracil
CMFVP	cyclophosphamide, methotrexate, fluorouracil, vincristine, prednisone
CMG	cystometrogram
CMHC	Community Mental Health Center
CMHN	Community Mental Health Nurse
CMI	cell-mediated immunity; Cornell Medical Index
CMJ	carpometacarpal joint
CMK	congenital multicystic kidney
CML	chronic myelogenous leukemia; cell-mediated lympholysis
CMM	cutaneous malignant melanoma
CMOPP	a drug combination protocol
CMRNG	chromosomally resistant Neisseria gonorrhoeae
$CMRO_2$	cerebral metabolic rate for oxygen
CMS	circulation motion sensation
CMSUA	clean midstream urinalysis
CMV	cytomegalovirus; cool mist vaporizer; controlled mechanical ventilation
CN	cranial nerve
Cn	cyanide
CNA	chart not available
CNCbl	cyanocobalamin
CNF	cyclophosphamide, mitoxantrone & fluorouracil
CNH	central neurogenic hypernea
CNM	certified nurse midwife
CNS	central nervous system; clinical nurse specialist
C/O	complained of; complaints; under care of
CO	cardiac output; carbon monoxide; castor oil
Co	cobalt
CO_2	carbon dioxide
CoA	coarctation of the aorta
COAD	chronic obstructive airway disease; chronic obstructive arterial disease
COAG	chronic open angle glaucoma
COAP	cyclophosphamide, vincristine, cytarabine and prednisone
COD	cause of death; codeine
COEPS	cortically originating extrapyramidal symptoms
COG	cognitive function tests; Central Oncology Group
COH	carbohydrate
COHB	carboxyhemoglobin
Coke	cocaine; Coca-Cola
Collyr	eye wash
col/ml	colonies per milliliter
COLD	chronic obstructive lung disease

COLD A	cold agglutin titer	CP	cerebral palsy; cleft palate; creatine phosphokinase; chest pain; chronic pain; chondromalacia patella
COMLA	a drug combination protocol		
COMP	complications; compound		
		C&P	cystoscopy and pyelography
COMT	catechol-o-methyl transferase	CPA	costophrenic angle; cerebellar pontile angle; cardiopulmonary arrest
CON A	concanavalin A		
conc.	concentrated		
CONG	congenital; gallon		
CONPA-DRI I	cyclophosphamide, vincristine, doxorubicin and melphalan	CPAF	chlorpropamide-alcohol flush
		CPAP	continuous positive airway pressure
CONPA-DRI II	conpadri I plus high-dose methotrexate	CPB	cardiopulmonary bypass
CONPA-DRI III	conpadri I plus intensified doxorubicin	CPBA	competitive protein-binding assay
COP	cycophosphamide, vincristine, prednisone; cicatricial ocular pemphigoid	CPC	clinicopathologic conference; cerebral palsy clinic
		CPCR	cardiopulmonary-cerebral resuscitation
COP-BLAM	a drug combination protocol	CPD	citrate-phosphate-dextrose; chorioretinopathy and pituitary dysfunction; cephalopelvic disproportion
COPD	chronic obstructive pulmonary disease		
COPE	chronic obstructive pulmonary emphysema		
COPP	cyclophosphamide, vincristine, procarbazine and prednisone	CPDD	calcium pyrophosphate deposition disease
		CPE	chronic pulmonary emphysema; cardiogenic pulmonary edema
cor	coronary		
COT	content of thought		
COTA	Certified Occupational Therapy Assistant	CPGN	chronic progressive glomerulonephritis
		CPH	chronic persistent hepatitis
COTX	cast off to x-ray		
COU	cardiac observation unit	CPI	constitutionally psychopathia inferior

CPID	chronic pelvic inflammatory disease	CR	cardiorespiratory; controlled release; cardiac rehabilitation; colon resection; closed reduction; complete remission
CPK	creatinine phosphokinase (BB, MB, MM are isoenzymes)		
CPKD	childhood polycystic kidney disease	CRA	central retinal artery
CPL	criminal procedure law	CRAO	central retinal artery occlusion
CPM	central pontine myelinolysis; cyclophosphamide; chlorpheniramine maleate; continuous passive motion; continue present management; counts per minute	CRBBB	complete right bundle branch block
		CRC	colorectal cancer
		CrCl	creatinine clearance
		CRD	chronic renal disease
		CREST	calcinosis, Raynaud's phenomenon, esophageal dysmotility, sclerodactyly, and telangiectasia
CPmax	peak serum concentration		
CPmin	trough serum concentration	CRF	chronic renal failure; corticotropin-releasing factor
CPN	chronic pyelonephritis		
CPP	cerebral perfusion pressure	CRI	chronic renal insufficiency
CPPB	continuous positive pressure breathing	CRIE	crossed radio-immuno-electro-phoresis
CPPD	cisplatin; calcium pyrophosphate dihydrate	crit.	hematocrit
CPPV	continuous positive pressure ventilation	CRL	crown rump length
CPR	cardiopulmonary resuscitation	CRNA	Certified Registered Nurse Anesthetist
CPS	complex partial seizures	CRNI	Certified Registered Nurse Intravenous
CPT	chest physio-therapy	CRNP	Certified Registered Nurse Practitioner
CPTH	chronic post-traumatic headache	CRO	cathode ray oscilloscope
CPZ	chlorpromazine; Compazine® (this is a dangerous abbreviation)	CRP	C-reactive protein
		CRPF	chloroquine-resistant plasmodium falciparum

CRST	calcification, Raynaud's phenomenom, scleroderma, and telangiectasia	CS IV	clinical stage 4
		CSLU	chronic status leg ulcer
CRT	copper reduction test; cathode ray tube; central reaction time	CSM	circulation, sensation, movement; cerebrospinal meningitis
Cr Tr	crutch training	CSOM	chronic serous otitis media
CRTT	Certified Respiratory Therapy Technician	CSP	cellulose sodium phosphate
CRTX	cast removed take x-ray	CSR	central supply room; Cheyne-Strokes respiration; corrective septorhinoplasty
CRVO	central retinal vein occlusion		
CS	cycloserine; clinical stage; consciousness; cat scratch; conjunctiva-sclera	CST	convulsive shock therapy; contraction stress test; cosyntropin stimulation test
C&S	culture and sensitivity	CSU	cardiac surveillance unit; cardiovascular surgery unit
C/S	cesarean section; culture and sensitivity		
CsA	cyclosporin	CT	computed tomography; circulation time; coagulation time; clotting time; corneal thickness; cervical traction; Coomb's test; cardiothoracic; calcitonin
CSB	caffeine sodium benzoate		
CSBF	coronary sinus blood flow		
CSC	cornea, sclera, conjunctiva		
CSD	cat scratch disease	Cta	catamenia (menses)
CSE	cross-section echocardiography	CTB	ceased to breathe
C sect.	cesarean section	CT & DB	cough, turn & deep breath
C-Sh	chair shower	CTD	chest tube drainage
CSH	carotid sinus hypersensitivity	CTF	Colorado tick fever
		CTL	cytotoxic T lymphocytes
CSF	cerebrospinal fluid; colony-stimulating factor	CTM	Chlor-Trimeton®
		CT/MPR	computed tomography with multiplanar reconstructions
CSICU	cardiac surgery intensive care unit		
CSII	continuous subcutaneous insulin infusion	cTNM	clinical-diagnostic staging of cancer

CTP	comprehensive treatment plan	CVP	central venous pressure; a drug combination protocol
CTR	carpal tunnel release		
CTS	carpal tunnel syndrome	CVRI	coronary vascular resistance index
CTSP	called to see patient		
CTW	central terminal of Wilson	CVS	clean voided specimen; chorionic villus sampling
CTX	cyclophosphamide (Cytoxan®)		
		CVUG	cysto-void urethrogram
CTXN	contraction		
CTZ	chemoreceptor trigger zone	C/W	consistent with; crutch walking
Cu	copper	CWE	cottonwool exudates
CU	cause unknown	CWMS	color, warmth, movement sensation
CUC	chronic ulcerative colitis		
		CWP	coal worker's pneumoconiosis
CUD	cause undetermined		
CUG	cystourethrogram	CWS	cotton wool spots
CUS	chronic undifferentiated schizophrenia	Cx	cervix; culture; cancel
		CxMT	cervical motion tenderness
CUSA	Cavitron ultrasonic aspirator		
		CXR	chest x-ray
CV	cardiovascular; cell volume	CyA	cyclosporine
		CYT	cyclophosphamide
CVA	cerebrovascular accident; costovertebral angle	Cyclo C	cyclocytidine HCl
		CYSTO	cystogram; cystoscopy
CVAT	costovertebral angle tenderness	CY-VA-DIC	cyclophosphamide, vincristine, adriamycin, dacarbazine
CVC	central venous catheter		
CVD	collagen vascular disease	CZI	crystalline zinc insulin (regular insulin)
CVI	cerebrovascular insufficiency; continuous venous infusion	CZN	chlorzotocin
CVID	common variable immune deficiency		

D

D	diarrhea; cholecalciferol; day; divorced; distal; dead; diopter
D_1, D_2	dorsal vertebra #1, #2

CVO	central vein occlusion; conjugate diameter of pelvic inlet

DA	dopamine; direct admission	DCH	delayed cutaneous hypersensitivity
DACT	dactinomycin	DCMXT	dichloromethotrexate
DAD	drug administration device	DCNU	chlorozotocin
DAG	dianhydrogalactitol	DCO	diffusing capacity of carbon monoxide
DAI	diffuse axonal injury	DCP®	calcium phosphate, dibasic
DAH	disordered action of the heart		
DAL	drug analysis laboratory	DCR	delayed cutaneous reaction
DAM	diacetylmonoxime	DCSA	double contrast shoulder arthrography
DANA	drug induced antinuclear antibodies	DCT	direct (antiglobulin) Coombs test; deep chest therapy
DAT	direct agglutination test; diet as tolerated; daunorubicin, cytarabine (ARA-C) and thioguanine; dementia of the Alzheimer type	DCTM	delay computer tomographic myelography
		DD	differential diagnosis; down drain; dependent drainage; dry dressing; Duchenne's dystrophy
DAW	dispense as written		
dB	decibel		
DB	date of birth	D & D	diarrhea and dehydration
DB & C	deep breathing and coughing	DDAVP®	desmopressin acetate
DBD	milolactol (dibromodulicitol)	DDD	degenerative disc disease
DBE	deep breathing exercise	DDP	cisplatin
DBED	Penicillin G benzathine	DDS	dialysis disequilibrium syndrome; doctor of dental surgery; 4, 4-diaminodiphenylsulfone (dapsone)
DBI®	phenformin HCl		
DBIL	direct bilirubin		
DBP	diastolic blood pressure		
DBQ	debrisoquin	DDST	Denver Development Screening Test
DBS	diminished breath sounds		
		DDT	chlorophenothane
DBZ	dibenzamine	DDx	differential diagnosis
D&C	dilation and curettage	D&E	dilation and evacuation
d/c, DC	discharged; discontinue; decrease; diagonal conjugate	DEC	decrease; diethylcarbamazine
		decub	decubitus
DC65®	Darvon Compound 65®	DEET	diethyltoluamide

28

DEF	decayed, extracted or filled	DHBV	duck hepatitis B virus
degen	degenerative	DHE 45®	dihydroergotamine mesylate
del	delivery, delivered		
DEP ST SEG	depressed ST segment	DHEA	dehydroepiandrosterone
		DHF	dengue hemorrhagic fever
DER	disulfiram-ethanol reaction	DHL	diffuse histocytic lymphoma
DES	disequilibrium syndrome; diethylstilbestrol; diffuse esophageal spasm	DHS	duration of hospital stay; Department of Human Services
DET	diethyltryptamine	DHT	dihydrotachysterol
DEV	duck embryo vaccine; deviation	DI	diabetes insipidus; detrusor instability
DEVR	dominant exudative vitreoretinopathy	diag.	diagnosis
		Diath SW	diathermy short wave
dex.	dexter (right)	DIC	disseminated intravascular coagulation; dacarbazine; Drug Information Center
DF	decayed and filled		
DFD	defined formula diets, diisopropyl phosphorofluoridate		
		DIE	die in emergency department
DFE	distal femoral epiphysis		
DFMC	daily fetal movement count	DIFF	differential blood count
		DIG	digoxin (this is a dangerous abbreviation)
DFO	deferoxamine		
DFOM	deferoxamine	DIJOA	dominantly inherited juvenile optic atrophy
DFP	isoflurophate (diisopropyl flurophosphate)		
		dil.	dilute
DFR	diabetic floor routine	DILD	diffuse infiltrative lung disease
DFU	dead fetus in uterus		
DGI	disseminated gonococcal infection	DILE	drug induced lupus erythematosus
DGM	ductal glandular mastectomy	DIM	diminish
		DIMOAD	diabetes insipidus, diabetes mellitus, optic atrophy and deafness
DH	developmental history; delayed hypersensitivity; diaphragmatic hernia		
		DIP	distal interphalangeal; desquamative interstitial pneumonia; drip infusion pyelogram
DHA	docosahexaenoic acid; dihydroxyacetone		
DHAD	mitoxanthrone HCl	dis.	dislocation

DIS	Diagnostic Interview Schedule (questionnaire)	DMO	dimethadone
disch.	discharge	DMOOC	diabetes mellitus out of control
DISH	diffuse idiopathic skeletal hyperostosis	DMSO	dimethyl sulfoxide
dist.	distilled	DMT	dimethyltryptamine
DIV	double inlet ventricle	DMV	Doctor of Veterinary Medicine
DIVA	digital intravenous angiography	DMX	diathermy, massage and exercise
DJD	degenerative joint disease	DN	down
DK	diabetic ketoacidosis; dark	DNA	deoxyribonucleic acid
DKA	diabetic ketoacidosis	DNCB	dinitrochlorobenzene
dl	deciliter (100 ml)	DNI	do not intubate
DL	danger list; deciliter; direct laryngoscopy; diagnostic laparoscopy	DNKA	did not keep appointment
		DNP	do not publish
DLE	discoid lupus erythematosus	DNR	do not resuscitate; do not report
DLMP	date of last menstrual period	DNS	do not show; deviated nasal septum; dysplastic nevus syndrome
DLNMP	date of last normal menstrual period		
D5LR	dextrose 5% in lactated Ringer's injection	D_5NSS	5% dextrose in normal saline solution
DM	diabetes mellitus; diastolic murmur; dextromethorphan; dermatomyositis	DO	osteopathic physician
		D/O	disorder
		DOA	dead on arrival; date of admission
DMBA	dimethylbenzantracene	DOA-DRA	dead on arrival despite resuscitative attempts
DMD	Doctor of Dental Medicine; Duchenne's muscular dystrophy	DOB	dobutamine; doctor's order book; date of birth
DME	durable medical equipment	DOC	died of other causes; diabetes out of control
DMF	decayed, missing or filled	DOCA	desoxycorticosterone acetate
DMI	desipramine	DOE	dyspnea on exertion
DMKA	diabetes mellitus ketoacidosis	DOH	Department of Health
		DOI	date of injury
		DOLV	double outlet left ventricle
		DON	Director of Nursing

DOP	dopamine	DRG	diagnosis-related groups
DORV	double-outlet right ventricle	DRSG	dressing
DORx	date of treatment	D/S	5% dextrose and 0.9% sodium chloride injection
DOSS	docusate sodium (dioctyl sodium sulfosuccinate)		
DOT	Doppler ophthalmic test; died on table	DS	double strength; disoriented; dextrose stick; discharge summary; Down's syndrome
DP	dorsalis pedis (pulse); diastolic pressure		
DPA	Department of Public Assistance	D5S	dextrose 5% in saline
DPC	discharge planning coordinator; delayed primary closure	DSA	digital subtraction angiography; (angiocardiography)
DPDL	diffuse poorly differentiated lymphocytic lymphoma	DSD	dry sterile dressing; discharge summary dictated
2,3-DPG	2,3-diphosphoglyceric acid	dsg	dressing
DPH	phenytoin (diphenylhydantoin); diphenhydramine; Department of Public Health; Doctor of Public Health	DSI	deep shock insulin
		DSM	drink skim milk
		DSM III	Diagnostic & Statistical Manual, 3rd Edition
DPM	Doctor of Podiatric Medicine; distintegrations per minute	DSS	dengue shock syndrome; docusate sodium
DPT	diphtheria, pertussis, tetanus (immunization); Demerol®, Phenergan® and Thorazine® (this is a dangerous abbreviation)	DST	dexamethasone suppression test; donor specific transfusion
		DT	discharge tomorrow; diphtheria tetanus; diphtheria toxoid; delirium tremens
DPV	delayed pressure urticaria		
Dr.	doctor	DTBC	tubocurarine (d-tubocurarine)
D.R.	delivery room; diabetic retinopathy	DTD #30	dispense 30 such doses
		DTH	delayed-type hypersensitivity
DREZ	dorsal root entry zone	DTIC	dacarbazine

31

DTPA	pentetic acid (di-ethylenetriamine-pentaacetic acid)	DYF	drag your feet
		Dz	disease; dozen
DTR	deep tendon reflexes		
DTs	delirium tremens		**E**
DTS	donor specific transfusion	E	edema
		4E	4 plus edema
DTT	diphtheria tetanus toxoid	E→A	say E,E,E, comes out as A,A,A upon auscultation of lung showing consolidation
DTV	due to void		
DTX	detoxification		
DU	duodenal ulcer; duroxide uptake; diabetic urine; diagnosis undetermined	EAA	electrothermal atomic absorption
		EAC	external auditory canal
		EACA	aminocaproic acid
DUB	dysfunctional uterine bleeding; Dubowitz (score)	EAHF	eczema, allergy, hay fever
		EAM	external auditory meatus
DUI	driving under the influence	EAST	external rotation, abduction stress test
dur	duration	EAT	ectopic atrial tachycardia
DVA	vindesine		
DVD	dissociated vertical deviation	EB	epidermolysis bullosa
		EBL	estimated blood loss
DVIU	direct vision internal urethrotomy	EBV	Epstein-Barr virus
		EC	enteric coated; eyes closed; extracellular
DVR	double valve replacement		
		ECA	ethacrynic acid
DVT	deep vein thrombosis	ECBD	exploration of common bile duct
D$_5$W	5% dextrose in water injection		
		ECC	emergency cardiac care; endocervical curettage
DW	dextrose in water; distilled water; deionized water		
		ECCE	extracapsular cataract extraction
5 DW	5% dextrose in water for injection	ECD	endocardial cushion defect
DWDL	diffuse well differentiated lymphocytic lymphoma		
		ECEMG	evoked compound electromyography
Dx	diagnosis	ECF	extracellular fluid; extended care facility
DXM	dexamethasone		

ECG	electrocardiogram	EDTA	edetic acid (ethylene-dinitrilo tetraacetic acid)
ECHO	etoposide, cyclophosphamide, Adriamycin®, vincristine; echocardiogram	EE	equine encephalitis; end to end
ECL	extend of cerebral lesion; extracapillary lesions	EEE	Eastern equine encephalomyelitis; edema, erythema and exudate
ECM	erythema chronicum migrans	EEG	electroencephalogram
ECMO	extracorporeal membrane oxygenation	EENT	eyes, ears, nose, throat
		EES®	erythromycin ethylsuccinate
ECN	extended care nursery	EF	extended-field (radiotherapy); endurance factor; ejection fraction
ECOG	Eastern Cooperative Oncology Group		
ECR	emergency chemical restraint	EFAD	essential fatty acid deficiency
ECRL	extensor carpi radialis longus	EFE	endocardial fibroelastosis
ECT	electroconvulsive therapy; enhanced computer tomography; emission computed tomography	EFM	external fetal monitoring
		EFW	estimated fetal weight
		e.g.	for example
ECU	extensor carpi ulnaris	EGA	estimated gestational age
ECW	extracellular water		
ED	emergency department; epidural	EGBUS	external genitalia, Bartholin, urethral, Skene's glands
ED$_{50}$	median effective dose		
EDC	estimated date of confinement; estimated date of conception; extensor digitorium communis; end diastolic counts	EGD	esophagogastroduodenoscopy
		EGTA	esophageal gastric tube airway
		EH	enlarged heart; essential hypertension; extramedullary hematopoiesis
EDD	expected date of delivery		
EDM	early diastolic murmur	EHDA	etidronate sodium
EDS	Ehler-Danlos syndrome	EHB	elevate head of bed
EDV	end-diastolic volume		

EHF	epidemic hemorrhagic fever
E & I	endocrine and infertility
EIA	exercise induced asthma
EIAB	extracranial-intra-cranial arterial bypass
EIB	exercise induced bronchospasm
EID	electronic infusion device
EIS	endoscopic injection scleropathy
EJ	external jugular; elbow jerk
EKG	electrocardiogram
EKC	epidemic keratocon-juctivitis
EKY	electrokymogram
E-L	external lids
ELF	elective low forceps
ELH	endolymphatic hydrops
ELISA	enzyme-linked immunosorbent assay
Elix	elixir
ELOP	estimated length of program
ELP	electrophoresis
EM	electron microscope; ejection murmur; erythema multiforme
EMB	ethambutol; endo-myocardial biopsy
EMC	encephalomyocarditis
EMD	electromechanical dis-sociation
EMF	erythrocyte maturation factor; evaporated milk formula
EMG	electromyograph; essential monoclonal gammopathy
EMIC	emergency maternity & infant care
E-MICR	electron microscopy
EMIT	enzyme multiplied immunoassay technique
EMR	emergency mechanical restraint; empty, mea-sure and record; edu-cable mentally retarded
EMS	emergency medical services
EMT	emergency medical technician
EMV	eye, motor, verbal (grading for Glasgow coma scale)
EMW	electromagnetic waves
ENA	extractable nuclear antigen
ENDO	endotracheal
ENG	electronystagmogram
ENL	erythema nodosum leprosum
ENP	extractable nucleo-protein
ENT	ears, nose, throat
EO	eyes open
EOA	examine, opinion, and advice; esophageal obturator airway
EOG	electro-oculogram; Ethrane®, oxygen and gas (nitrous oxide)
EOM	extraocular movement; extraocular muscles
EOMI	extraocular muscles intact

EORA	elderly onset rheumatoid arthritis		ERP	estrogen receptor protein; emergency room physician; endoscopic retrograde pancreatography
eos.	eosinophil			
EP	endogenous pyrogen; electrophysiologic			
EPA	eicosapentaenoic acid		ERPF	effective renal plasma flow
EPB	extensor pollicis brevis			
EPEG	etoposide		ERT	estrogen replacement therapy
EPI	epinephrine			
EPIS	episiotomy		ERV	expiratory reserve volume
epith.	epithelial			
EPL	extensor pollicis longus		ESAP	evoked sensory (nerve) action potention
EPM	electronic pacemaker			
EPP	erythropoietic protoporphyria		ESC	end systolic counts
			ESM	ejection systolic murmur
EPR	electrophrenic respiration		ESP	especially; end systolic pressure
ERA	evoked response audiometry			
			ESR	erythrocyte sedimentation rate
EPR	emergency physical restraint			
			ESRD	end-stage renal disease
			ess.	essential
EPS	electrophysiologic study; extrapyramidal syndrome (symptom)		EST	electroshock therapy
			ESWL	extracorporeal shock-wave lithotripsy
EPT®	early pregnancy test		ET	endotracheal; esotropia; eustachian tube; exercise treadmill; ejection time
EPTS	existed prior to service			
ER	emergency room; estrogen receptors; external rotation			
			et	and
			ETA	ethionamide
ERA	estrogen receptor assay		et al	and others
ERCP	endoscopic retrograde cholangiopancreatography		ETF	eustachian tubal function
			ETH	elixir terpin hydrate; ethanol
ERFC	erythrocyte rosette forming cells		ETHc̄C	elixir terpin hydrate with codeine
ERG	electroretinogram		EtO	ethylene oxide; estimated time of ovulation
ERL	effective refractory length			

ETOH	alcohol; alcoholic	FACA	Fellow of the American College of Anaesthetists
ETT	endotracheal tube; exercise tolerance test	FACAG	Fellow of the American College of Angiology
EU	excretory urography		
EUA	examine under anesthesia	FACAL	Fellow of the American College of Allergy
EVAC	evacuation	FACAN	Fellow of the American College of Anesthesiologists
eval	evaluate		
EWB	estrogen withdrawal bleeding	FACAS	Fellow of the American College of Abdominal Surgeons
EWSCLs	extended-wear soft contact lenses	FACC	Fellow of the American College of Cardiology
exam.	examination		
EXP	experienced; exploration	FACCP	Fellow of the American College of Chest Physicians
exp. lap.	exploratory laparotomy		
ext.	extract; external	FACCPC	Fellow of the American College of Clinical Pharmacology & Chemotherapy
ext. rot.	external rotation		
EX U	excretory urogram		

F

F	Fahrenheit; female; firm; flow; facial; French	FACD	Fellow of the American College of Dentists
F_1	offspring from the first generation	FACGE	Fellow of the American College of Gastroenterology
F_2	offspring from the second generation		
FA	folic acid; femoral artery	FACH	forceps to after-coming head
FAAP	family assessment adjustment pass	FACLM	Fellow of the American College of Legal Medicine
FAB	French-American-British Cooperative group	FACN	Fellow of the American College of Nutrition
FAC	fluorouracil, Adriamycin®, cyclophosphamide; fractional area concentration	FACNP	Fellow of the American College of Neuropsychopharmacology

FACOG	Fellow of the American College of Obstetricians & Gynecologists	FB	fasting blood sugar; finger breadth; foreign body
FACOS	Fellow of the American College of Orthopedic Surgeons	FBH	hydroxybutyric dehydrogenase
FACP	Fellow of the American College of Physicians	FBS	fasting blood sugar; fetal bovine serum
FACPRM	Fellow of the American College of Preventive Medicine	FBU	fingers below umbilicus
		FBW	fasting blood work
		FC	foley catheter; finger counting
FACR	Fellow of the American College of Radiology	5-FC	flucytosine
		FC	fever, chills
FACS	Fellow of the American College of Surgeons	F + C	flare and cells
		F & C	foam and condom
FACSM	Fellow of the American College of Sports Medicine	F. cath.	foley catheter
		FCC	follicular center cells; familial colonic cancer; fracture compound comminuted
FAD	Family Accessment Device		
FAI	functional assessment inventory	FCDB	fibrocystic disease of the breast
FALL	fallopian	FCH	familial combined hyperlipidemia
FAM	fluorouracil, Adriamycin, mitomycin; family	FCMC	family centered maternity care
FANA	fluorescent antinuclear antibody	FCMD	Fukiyama's congenital muscular dystrophy
FAP	fibrillating action potential; familial amyloid polyneuropathy	FCMN	family centered maternity nursing
		FCR	flexor carpi radialis
		FCRB	flexor carpi radialis brevis
FAS	fetal alcohol syndrome	FCSNVD	fever, chills, sweating, nausea, vomiting, diarrhea
FAST	fluoro-allergo sorbent test		
		FCU	flexor carpi ulnaris
FAT	fluorescent antibody test	FD	focal distance; familial dysautonomia
		F & D	fixed and dilated

FDA	Food and Drug Administration; fronto-dextra anterior	FHI	Fuch's heterochromic iridocyclitis
FDIU	fetal death in utero	FHR	fetal heart rate
FDP	fibrin-degradation products; flexor digitorum profundus	FHS	fetal heart sounds
		FHT	fetal heart tone
FDS	flexor digitorum superficialis; for duration of stay	FIGLU	formiminoglutamic acid
		$FiCO_2$	fraction of inspired carbon dioxide
Fe, fe	iron; female	FIGO	International Federation of Gynecology and Obstetrics
FEC	forced expiratory capacity		
FEF	forced expiratory flow rate	FiO_2	fraction of inspired oxygen
FEL	familial erythrophagocytic lymphohistiocytosis	FITC	fluorescein isothiocynate
		FL	fluid
		FLK	funny looking kid
FEM	femoral	FLS	flashing lights and/or scotoma
Fem-pop	femoral popliteal (bypass)		
FEN	fluid, electrolytes, nutrition	FM	fetal movements; face mask
		F & M	firm and midline (uterus)
FENa	fractional extraction of sodium		
		FMC	fetal movement count
FEP	free erythrocyte protoporphorin	FMD	foot and mouth disease; family medical doctor
$FeSO_4$	ferrous sulfate		
FEV_1	forced expiratory volume in one second	FME	full mouth extraction
		FMF	familial Mediterranean fever; forced midexpiratory flow
FF	filtration fraction; fundus firm; flat feet; fat free; force fluids		
		FMG	foreign medical graduate; fine mesh gauze
FFA	free fatty acid		
FFP	fresh frozen plasma	FMH	fibromuscular hyperplasia
FFT	fast-Fourier transforms		
FH	family history; fetal heart; fundal height	$FML^®$	fluorometholone
		FMP	fasting metabolic panel
FHF	fulminant hepatic failure	FMX	full mouth x-ray
FHH	familial hypocalciuric hypercalcemia	FN	finger-to-nose; false negative

38

F to N	finger to nose	FPNA	first-pass nuclear angiocardiography
FNAB	fine-needle aspiration biopsy	FPZ	fluphenazine
FNAC	fine-needle aspiratory cytology	FPZ-D	fluphenazine decanoate
		FR	flow rate
FNCJ	fine needle catheter jejunostomy	F & R	force & rhythm (pulse)
FNH	focal nodular hyperplasia	FRC	functional residual capacity
FNR	false negative rate	FRJM	full range of joint motion
FNS	functional neuromuscular stimulation	FROM	full range of movement
FOB	foot of bed; fiberoptic bronchoscope; father of baby	FS	frozen section; flexible sigmoidoscopy
		FSB	fetal scalp blood
FOBT	fecal occult blood test	FSBM	full strength breast milk
FOC	father of child	FSE	fetal scalp electrode
FOD	free of disease	FSG	focal & segmental glomerulosclerosis
FOG	Fluothane®, oxygen and gas (nitrous oxide)	FSH	follicle stimulating hormone; facioscapulo-humeral
FOI	flight of ideas		
FOMi	fluorouracil, Oncovin (vincristine), and mitomycin	FSHMD	facioscapulohumeral muscular dystrophy
FOOB	fell out of bed	FSP	fibrin split products
FOI	flight of ideas	FSS	French steel sound (dilated to #24FSS)
F.P.	family planning; false positive; flat plate; frozen plasma; family practice	ft.	foot
		FT	full term
		FT$_3$	free triiodorhyroxine
fpA	fibrinopeptide A	FT$_4$	free thyroxine
F.P.A.L.	fullterm, premature, abortion, living	F$_3$T	trifluridine
FPB	flexor pollicis brevis	FTA	fluorescent titer antibody; fluorescent treponemal antibody
FPD	feto-pelvic dispro-portion; fixed partial denture	FTD	failure to descend
		FTI	free thyroxine index
FPG	fasting plasma glucose	FTLFC	full term living female child
FPIA	fluorescence-polariza-tion immunoassay	FTLMC	full term living male child
FPL	flexor pollicis longus		

FTN	finger-to-nose; full term nursery		GA	gastric analysis; glucose/acetone; general appearance; general anesthesia; gestational age
FTND	full-term normal delivery			
FTP	failure to progress		GABA	gamma-aminobutyric acid
FTR	for the record			
F.T.S.G.	full-thickness skin graft		GABHS	group A beta hemolytic streptococci
FTT	failure to thrive			
F & U	flanks and upper quadrants		GAG	glycosaminoglycan
			GAS	general adaption syndrome
F/U	follow-up; fundus at umbilicus			
			GAT	group adjustment therapy
F↑U	finger above umbilicus			
F↓U	finger below umbilicus		GB	gallbladder
5-FU	fluorouracil		GBH	gamma benzene hexachloride (lindane)
FUB	function uterine bleeding			
			GBM	glomerular basement membrane
FUDR®	floxuridine			
FUN	follow-up note		GBP	gastric bypass
FUO	fever of undetermined origin		GBS	gallbladder series; Guillain-Barre syndrome; group B streptococci
FVC	forced vital capacity			
FVH	focal vascular headache			
FVL	flow volume loop		GC	gonococci (gonorrhea); geriatric chair (Gerichair)
FWB	full weight bearing			
FWW	front wheel walker			
Fx	fracture; fractional urine		G−C	gram-negative cocci
			G+C	gram-positive cocci
Fx-dis	fracture-dislocation		GCDFP	gross cystic disease fluid protein
FXN	function			
FXR	fracture		GCIIS	glucose control insulin infusion system
			GCS	Glasgow coma scale
			GCT	giant cell tumor
			GD	Graves' disease

G

G	gauge; gravida; gram; gallop		G and D	growth and development
			GDF	gel diffusion precipitin
G1-4	grade 1-4		GDM	gestational diabetes mellitus
G-11	hexachlorophene		GE	gastroenteritis

GENT	gentamicin	giv	given
GEP	gastroenteropancreatic	GJ	gastrojejunostomy
GER	gastroesophageal reflux	GL	greatest length
GERD	gastroesophageal reflux disease	GLA	gingivolinguoaxial
GETA	general endotracheal anesthesia	GLU 5	five hour glucose tolerance test
GF	grandfather; gluten-free; gastric fistula	GM	grandmother; gram
		GMP	guanosine mono-phosphate
GFR	glomerular filtration rate	GMTs	geometric mean antibody titers
GG	gamma globulin; guaifenesin	GN	graduate nurse; glomerulonephritis; gram negative
GGE	generalize glandular enlargement		
GGT	gamma-glutamyl trans-peptidase	GnRH	gonadotropin-releasing hormone
GGTP	gamma glutamyl trans-peptidase	GOG	Gynecologic Oncology Group
GH	growth hormone	GOK	God only knows
GHB	gamma hydroxy-butyrate	GOT	glutamic-oxaloacetic transaminase; aspartate aminotransferase; glucose oxidase test
GHb	glycosylated hemoglobin		
GHD	growth hormone deficiency	GP	general practitioner; gutta percha
GHQ	General Health Questionnaire	G/P	gravida/para
GI	gastrointestinal; granuloma inguinale	G_4P_{3104}	four pregnancies (gravid), 3 went to term, one premature, no abortion (or miscarriage) and 4 living children (p = para)
GIB	gastric ileal bypass		
GIC	general immuno-competence		
GIK	glucose-insulin-potassium	GPC	gram positive cocci; giant papillary conjunctivitis
GIP	giant cell interstitial pneumonia; gastric inhibitory peptide	G6PD	glucose-6-phosphate dehydrogenase
		GPMAL	gravida, para, multiple births, abortions and live births
GIS	gastrointestinal series		
GIT	gastrointestinal tract		
GITSG	Gastrointestinal Tumor Study Group	GPN	graduate practical nurse

GPT	glutamic pyruvic transaminase
gr	grain (approximately 60 mg) (this is a dangerous abbreviation)
G−R	gram-negative rods
G+R	gram-positive rods
Grav.	gravid (pregnant)
GRD	gastroesophageal reflux disease
GRN	granules
$Gr_1P_0AB_1$	one pregnancy, no births, one abortion
GSC	Glasgow coma scale
GSD	glucogen storage disease
GSD-1	glycogen storage disease, type 1
GSE	grip strong and equal; gluten sensitive enteropathy
GSI	genuine stress incontinence
GSP	general survey panel
GSPN	greater superficial petrosal neurectomy
GSR	galvanic skin resistance
GST	gold sodium thiomalate
GSTM	gold sodium thiomalate
GSW	gunshot wound
GT	gastrotomy tube; gait training
GTN	gestational trophoblastic neoplasms
GTP	glutamyl transpeptidase
GTT	glucose tolerance test; drop
GTT agar	gelatin-tellurite-taurocholate agar
GTTS	drops
GU	genitourinary
GUS	genitourinary sphincter; genitourinary system
GVF	good visual fields
GVHD	graft-versus-host disease
GWA	gunshot wound of the abdomen
GWT	gunshot wound of the throat
GXT	graded exercise testing
GYN	gynecology

H

H	hypodermic; hour; heroin; hydrogen; husband
3H	high, hot and a helluva lot
HA	headache; hyperalimentation; hypothalmic amenorrhea; hearing aid; hemolytic anemia; hospital admission
HAA	hepatitis-associated antigen
HAE	hereditary angioedema; hepatic artery embolization; hearing aid evaluation
HAI	hepatic arterial infusion
HAL	hyperalimentation
HAM-A	Hamilton Anxiety (scale)
HAM D	Hamilton Depression (scale)

HAN	heroin associated nephropathy	HBV	hepatitis B virus; hepatitis B vaccine; honeybee venom
HANE	hereditary angioneurotic edema	HC	hydrocortisone; home care; head circumference; Hickman catheter; house call
HAPS	hepatic arterial perfusion scintigraphy		
HAQ	Headache Assessment Questionnaire	HCA	health care aide
HAS	hyperalimentation solution	HCC	hepatocellular carcinoma
HASHD	hypertensive arteriosclerotic heart disease	HCG	human chorionic gonadotropin
HAT	head, arms & trunk	HCl	hydrochloric acid; hydrochloride
HAV	hepatitis A virus; hallux abducto valgus	HCL	hair cell leukemia
		HCLs	hard contact lenses
HB	hemoglobin; heart block; hold breakfast	HCM	health care maintenance; hypertropic cardiomyopathy
HBBW	hold breakfast blood work		
		HCO_3	bicarbonate
HBD	hydroxybutyric acid dehydrogenase; has been drinking	HCP	hereditary coporphyria
		HCT	hematocrit; hydrocortisone; histamine challenge test
HBGM	home blood glucose monitoring		
HBI	hemibody irradiation	HCTZ	hydrochlorothiazide
HBIG	hepatitis B immune globulin	HCVD	hypertensive cardiovascular disease
Hb Kansas	mutant hemoglobin with a low affinity for oxygen	HD	hearing distance; Hodgkin's disease; hemodialysis; helloma molle; hip disarticulation; high dose; Huntington's disease
HbA_{1c}	glycosylated hemoglobin		
HBF	hepatic blood flow		
HBO	hyperbaric oxygen	HDARAC	high dose cytarabine (ARA C)
HBP	high blood pressure	HDCV	human diploid cell vaccine
HBS	Health Behavior Scale		
HBsAg	hepatitis B surface antigen	HDL	high-density lipoprotein
HBSS	Hank's balanced salt solution	HDLW	hearing distance for watch in left ear

HDRW	hearing distance for watch in right ear	HH	hiatal hernia; home health; hypogonadotrophic hypogonadism; hard of hearing
HDMTX	high-dose methotrexate		
HDN	hemolytic disease of the newborn	H&H	hematocrit and hemoglobin
HDPAA	heparin-dependent platelet-associated antibody	HHC	home health care
		HHD	hypertensive heart disease
HDRS	Hamilton Depression Rate Scale	HHFM	high humidity face mask
H&E	hemorrhage and exudate; hematoxylin and eosin	HHN	hand held nebulizer
		HHNK	hyperglycemic hyperosmolar nonketotic (coma)
HEENT	head, eyes, ears, nose, throat		
HEK	human embryonic kidney	HHT	hereditary hemorrhagic telangiectasis
HEL	human embryonic lung	HI	hemagglutination inhibition; head injury
hemi	hemiplegia		
HEMPAS	hereditary erythrocytic multinuclearity with positive acidified serum test	HIA	hemagglutination inhibition antibody
		5-HIAA	5 hydroxyindolacetic acid
HEP	histamine equivalent prick; hepatic	HIB	Haemophilus influenzae type b (vaccine)
HES	hypereosinophilic syndrome	hi-cal	high caloric
Hex	hexamethylmelamine	HID	headache, insomnia, depression
HF	heart failure	HIDA	hepato-iminodiacetic acid (lidofenin)
HFD	high forceps delivery		
HFHL	high frequence hearing loss	HIE	hypoxic-ischemic encephalopathy
Hgb	hemoglobin	HIF	higher integrative functions
HGH	human growth hormone	HIL	hypoxic-ischemic lesion
HGPRT	hypoxanthine-guanine phosphoribosyltransferase	HIR	head injury routine
		HIS	Health Intention Scale
		Histo	histoplasmin skin test

HIT	heparin induced thrombocytopenia; histamine inhalation test	HMX	heat massage exercise
		HN	high nitrogen
		H&N	head and neck
		HN_2	mechlorethamine HCl
HIVD	herniated intervertebral disc	HNP	herniated nucleus pulposus
HJR	hepato-jugular reflex	HNRNA	heterogeneous nuclear ribonucleic acid
H-K	hand to knee		
HKAFO	hip-knee-ankle-foot orthosis	HNV	has not voided
		HO	house officer
HKO	hip-knee orthosis	H/O	history of
HL	hairline; heparin lock; hearing level; hallux limitus; harelip; Hickman line; haloperidol	H_2O	water
		H_2O_2	hydrogen peroxide
		HOB	head of bed
		HOB UPSOB	head of bed up for shortness of breath
HL-D	haloperidol decanoate		
HLA	human lymphocyte antigen	HOC	Health Officer Certificate
HLD	herniated lumbar disc	HOCM	hypertrophic obstructive cardiomyopathy
HLHS	hypoplastic left heart syndrome	HOG	halothane, oxygen and gas (nitrous oxide)
HLV	hypoplastic left ventricle	HOH	hard of hearing
HM	hand motion; human semisynthetic insulin	HOPI	history of present illness
HMB	homatropine methyl-bromide	HP	hemiplegia; hydrophilic petrolatum; hot packs; hemipelvectomy
HMD	hyaline membrane disease	H&P	history and physical
HMG	human menopausal gonadotropin	HPA	human papilloma virus; hypothalamic-pituitary-adrenal (axis)
HMG CoA	hepatic hydroxymeth-ylglutaryl coenzyme A		
HMI	healed myocardial infarction	HPF	high-power field
HMM	hexamethylmelamine	HPFH	hereditary persistence of fetal hemoglobin
HMO	Health Maintenance Organization	HPI	history of present illness
HMP	hexose monophos-phate; hot moist packs		
HMR	histocytic medullary reticulosis	HPL	human placenta lactogen

45

HPLC	high-pressure (performance) liquid chromatography	HSM	hepato-splenomegaly; holosystolic murmur
HPG	human pituitary gonadotropin	HSP	Henoch-Schönlein purpura
HPL	hyperplexia	HSR	heated serum reagin
HPM	hemiplegic migraine	HSSE	high soap suds enema
HPN	home parenteral nutrition	HSV	herpes simplex virus
HPO	hypertrophic pulmonary osteoarthropathy; hydrophilic ointment	HT	hubbard tank; hypertension; hypermetropia; height; heart; hammertoe; hyperopia
HPT	hyperparathyroidism	5-HT	5-hydroxytryptamine
HPZ	high pressure zone	ht. aer.	heated aerosol
HQC	hydroquinone cream	HTAT	human tetanus antitoxin
HR	heart rate; hour; hallux rigidus; Harrington rod; hospital record	HTC	hypertensive crisis
		HTF	house tube feeding
HRA	histamine releasing activity	HTL	human thymic leukemia
HRC	Human Rights Committee	HTLV III	human T cell lymphotrophic virus type III
HRLA	human reovirus-like agent	HTN	hypertension
		HTP	House-Tree-Person-test
HRP	horseradish peroxidase	5-HTP	5-hydroxytryptophan
HRS	hepatorenal syndrome	HTVD	hypertensive vascular disease
HS	bedtime; Hartman's solution (lactated Ringer's); hereditary spherocytosis; heel spur; heel stick; herpes simplex	HU	hydroxyurea
		HUIFM	human leukocyte interferon meloy
		HUR	hydroxyurea
		HUS	hemolytic uremic syndrome
H→S	heel to shin	HV	has voided; hallux valgus
HSA	human serum albumin; Health Systems Agency; hypersomnia-sleep apnea	H&V	hemigastrecotomy and vagotomy
		HVA	homovanillac acid
HSBG	heel stick blood gas	HW	heparin well; housewife
HSE	herpes simplex encephalitis	hwb	hot water bottle
HSG	histosalpingogram	Hx	history; hospitalization

HXM	hexamethylmelamine		IBC	iron binding capacity
Hz	Hertz		IBD	inflammatory bowel
HZ	herpes zoster			disease
HZO	herpes zoster ophthalmicus		IBI	intermittent bladder irrigation
			ibid	at the same place
			IBNR	incurred but not reported
I			IBS	irritable bowel syndrome
I	independent; impression; one; incisal		IBW	ideal body weight
I_2	iodine		IC	individual counseling; intracranial; irritable colon; intercostal
I^{131}	radioactive iodine			
IA	intra-amniotic		ICA	internal carotid artery
IAA	interrupted aortic arch		ICBT	intercostobronchial trunk
IABC	intra-aortic balloon counterpulsation		ICCE	intracapsular cataract extraction
IABP	intra-aortic balloon pump		ICCU	intermediate coronary care unit
IAC	internal auditory canal		ICD	isocitrate dehydrogenase; instantaneous cardiac death
IAC-CPR	interposed abdominal compressions—cardiopulmonary resuscitation			
IACP	intra-aortic counterpulsation		ICD 9 CM	International Classification of Diseases, 9th Revision, Clinical Modification
IA DSA	intra-arterial subtraction arteriography			
IAHA	immune adherence hemagglutination		ICF	intracellular fluid; intermediate care facility
IAI	intra-abdominal infection			
IAM	internal auditory meatus		ICG	indocyanine green
			ICH	intranial hemorrhage
IAN	intern admission note		ICM	intracostal margin
IAP	intermittent acute porphyria		ICN	intensive care nursery
			ICP	intracranial pressure
IASD	interatrial septal defect		ICPP	intubated continuous positive pressure
IAT	indirect antiglobulin test		ICRF-159	razoxane
IB	isolation bed		ICS	intracostal space

ICSH	interstitial cell-stimulating hormone	IF	intrinsic factor; involved field (radiotherapy); interferon; immunofluorescence
ICT	intensive conventional therapy; inflammation of connective tissue	IFA	indirect fluorescent antibody test
ICU	intensive care unit	IFN	interferon
ICVH	ischemic cerebrovascular headache	IgA	immunoglobulin A
ICW	intercellular water	IgD	immunoglobulin D
ID	intradermal; initial dose; infectious disease (physician or department); identification; immunodiffusion; the same; identify	IgE	immunoglobulin E
		IgG	immunoglobulin G
		IGIV	immune globulin intravenous
		IgM	immunoglobulin M
I & D	incision and drainage	IGR	intrauterine growth retardation
IDE	Investigational Device Exemption	IGT	impaired glucose tolerance
IDDM	insulin-dependent diabetes mellitus	IH	infectious hepatitis; indirect hemagglutination; inguinal hernia
IDDS	implantable drug delivery system	IHA	indirect hemagglutination
IDFC	immature dead female child	IHC	immobilization hypercalcemia
IDM	infant of a diabetic mother	IHD	ischemic heart disease; intraheptic duct (ule)
IDMC	immature dead male child	IHH	idiopathic hypogonadotrophic hypogonadism
IDS	Infectious Disease Service		
IDU	idoxuridine	IHS	Iodiopathic Headache Score
IDV	intermittent demand ventilation	IHs	iris hamartomas
i.e.	that is	IHSS	idiopathic hypertrophic subaortic stenosis
IEC	inpatient exercise center	IHT	insulin hypoglycemia test
IEF	iso-electric focusing		
IEM	immune electron microscopy	IICP	increased intracranial pressure
IEP	individualized education program; immunoelectrophoresis	IICU	infant intensive care unit

IJ	internal jugular; ileojejunal	INDM	infant of nondiabetic mother
IL	Intralipid®; interleukin (1, 2, and 3)	INEX	inexperienced
ILD	ischemic leg disease	INF	inferior; infusion; infant; infected
ILFC	immature living female child	ING	inguinal
ILM	internal limiting membrane	INH	isoniazid
		inj	injection; injury
ILMC	immature living male child	INS	insurance
		INST	instrumental delivery
ILMI	inferolateral myocardial infarct	int.	internal
		int-rot	internal rotation
IM	intramuscular; infectious mononucleosis; intermetatarsal; internal medicine	inver	inversion
		I&O	intake and output
		IO	intraocular pressure; inferior oblique; initial opening
IMA	inferior mesenteric artery; internal mammary artery	IOC	intern on call; intraoperative cholangiogram
IMAG	internal mammary artery graft	IOD	interorbital distance
		IOF	intraocular fluid
IMB	intermenstrual bleeding	IOFB	intraocular foreign body
IMF	intermaxillary fixation	IOH	idiopathic orthostatic hypotension
IMG	internal medicine group (group practices)	IOL	intraocular lens
IMH test	indirect microhemagglutination test	ION	ischemic optic neuropathy
IMI	inferior myocardial infarction; imipramine	IOP	intraocular pressure
		IORT	intraoperative radiation therapy
IMIG	intramuscular immunoglobulin	IOS	intraoperative sonography
IMN	internal mammary (lymph) node	IOV	initial office visit
IMP	impression; impacted	IP	intraperitoneal
IMV	intermittent mandatory ventilation	IPA	isopropyl alcohol; invasive pulmonary aspergillosis
INC	incontinent; incomplete; inside-the-needle catheter	IPCD	infantile polycystic disease
IND	investigational new drug		

IPD	immediate pigment darkening; intermittent peritoneal dialysis	ISDN	isosorbide dinitrate
IPFD	intrapartum fetal distress	ISG	immune serum globulin
		ISH	isolated systolic hypertension
IPG	individually polymerized grass	ISMA	infantile spinal muscular atrophy
IPJ	interphalangeal joint	ISO	isoproterenol
IPK	intractable plantar keratosis	ISS	Injury Severity Score
IPMI	inferoposterior myocardial infarct	IST	insulin sensitivity test; insulin shock therapy
IPN	infantile periarteritis nodosa; intern's progress note	ISW	interstitial water
		IT	intrathecal; inhalation therapy; intertuberous
IPP	inflatable penile prosthesis	ITCP	idiopathic thrombocytopenia purpura
IPPA	inspection, palpation, percussion and auscultation	ITE	insufficient therapeutic effect
		ITP	idiopathic thrombocytopenic purpura; interim treatment plan
IPPB	intermittent positive pressure breathing		
IPPV	intermittent positive pressure ventilation	ITVAD	indwelling transcutaneous vascular access device
IPV	inactivated polio vaccine	IU	international unit
IQ	intelligence quotient	IUD	intrauterine device; intrauterine death
IR	infrared; internal rotation	IUFD	intrauterine fetal death
IRBBB	incomplete right bundle branch block	IUGR	interuterine growth retardation
IRMA	intraretinal microvascular abnormalities	IUP	intrauterine pregnancy
		IUPD	intrauterine pregnancy delivered
IRR	intrarenal reflux	IV	intravenous; four; symbol for class 4 controlled substances
IRV	inspiratory reserve volume		
IS	intercostal space; incentive spirometer; induced sputum	IVA	Intervir-A
		IVC	intravenous cholangiogram; inferior vena cava; intraventricular catheter
ISB	incentive spirometry breathing		
ISCs	irreversible sickle cells	IVD	intravenous drip; intervertebral disk

IVF	*in vitro* fertilization; intravenous fluid(s)		JODM	juvenile onset diabetes mellitus
IVFE	intravenous fat emulsion		JP	Jobst pump; Jackson-Pratt (drain)
IVGTT	intravenous glucose tolerance test		JRA	juvenile rheumatoid arthritis
IVH	intravenous hyperali-mentation; intraven-tricular hemorrhage		jt	joint
			juv.	juvenile
IVIG	intravenous immuno-globulin		JVD	jugular venous disten-tion
IVLBW	infant of very low birth weight		JVP	jugular venous pulse; jugular venous pressure
IVP	intravenous pyelogram; intravenous push		JVPT	jugular venous pulse tracing
IVPB	intravenous piggyback			
IVR	idioventricular rhythm			
IVS	intraventricular septum			

K

IVSD	intraventricular septal defect		K	potassium; vitamin K
IVSS	intravenous Soluset		K_1	phytonadione
IVU	intravenous urography		K_3	menadione
IWL	insensible water loss		K_4	menadiol sodium diphosphate
IWMI	inferior wall myo-cardial infarct		KA	ketoacidosis
			KAFO	knee-ankle-foot orthosis

J

			KAO	knee-ankle orthosis
J	Jewish; joint		KAS	Katz Adjustment Scale
JAMG	juvenile autoimmune myasthenia gravis		K Cal	kilocalorie
			KCl	potassium chloride
JC	junior clinicians (medi-cal students)		KCS	keratoconjunctivitis sicca
JDMS	juvenile dermato-myositis		KD	Kawasaki's disease; Keto Diastex®; knee disarticulation
JE	Japanese encephalitis			
JF	joint fluid		KDA	known drug allergies
JI	jejunoileal		KF	kidney function
JIB	jejunoileal bypass		KFD	Kyasanur Forrest disease
JJ	jaw jerk			
JMS	junior medical student		kg	kilogram
jnt	joint		K24H	potassium, urine 24 hour

KI	potassium iodide; karyopyknotic index	L + A	light and accommodation
KID	keratitis, ichthyosis and deafness (syndrome)	Lab	laboratory
		LAC	laceration; long arm cast
KILO	kilogram	LAD	left anterior descending; left axis deviation
KISS	saturated solution of potassium iodide	LAD-MIN	left axis deviation minimal
KJ	knee jerk		
KK	knee kick	LAE	left atrial enlargement
KLH	keyhole limpet hemocyanin	LAF	Latin-American female; lymphocyte-activating factor; laminar air flow
KM	kanamycin		
KMnO₄	potassium permanganate	LAG	lymphangiogram
		LAL	left axillary line; limulus amebocyte lysate
KNO	keep needle open		
KO	keep open	LAM	Latin-American male
KOH	potassium hydroxide	LAN	lymphadenopathy
KP	keratoprecipitate; hot pack	LAO	left anterior oblique
		LAP	laparotomy; laparoscopy; leucine amino peptidase; left arterial pressure; leukocyte alkaline phosphatase
KS	Kaposi's sarcoma		
17-KS	17-ketosteroids		
KTU	kidney transplant unit		
KUB	kidney, ureter, bladder		
KVO	keep vein open		
KW	Keith-Wagener (ophthalmoscopic finding, graded I-IV); Kimmelstiel-Wilson	LAPMS	long arm posterior molded splint
		LAS	leucine acetylsalicylate
		L-ASP	asparaginase
		LAT	lateral; left anterior thigh
KWB	Keith, Wagener, Barker	LATS	long-acting thyroid stimulator
K-wire	Kirschner wire		
		LAV	lymphadenopathy associated virus

L

L	left; liter; lente insulin; fifty; lumbar; lingual	LB	low back; left breast; pound; left buttock; large bowel
L₂	second lumbar vertebra		
LA	left atrium; local anesthesia; long acting; Latin American; left arm	LBB	left breast biopsy
		LBBB	left bundle branch block
		LBCD	left border of cardiac dullness

LBD	left border dullness	LD	lethal dose; liver disease; lactic dehydrogenase (formerly LDH); loading dose; labor and delivery; levodopa
LBM	lean body mass; loose bowel movement		
LBO	large bowel obstruction		
LBP	low back pain; low blood pressure		
LBV	left brachial vein	LDB	Legionnaires disease bacterium
LBW	low birth weight		
LC	living children; low calorie	LDDS	local dentist
		LDH	lactic dehydrogenase
LCA	left coronary artery; Leber's congenital amaurosis	LDL	low-density lipoprotein
		LDV	laser Doppler velocimetry
LCAT	lecithin cholesterol acyltransferase	LE	lupus erythematosus; lower extremities
LCCA	leukocytoclastic angiitis; left common carotid artery	LED	lupus erythematosus disseminatus
		LEHPZ	lower esophageal high pressure zone
LCCS	low cervical cesarean section	L-ERX	leukoerythroblastic reaction
LCD	coal tar solution (liquor carbonis detergens); localized collagen dystrophy	LES	lower esophageal sphincter; local excitatory state
		LESP	lower esophageal sphincter pressure
LCGU	local cerebral glucose utilization	LET	linear energy transfer
LCH	local city hospital	LF	low forceps; left foot
LCLC	large cell lung carcinoma	LFA	left fronto-anterior; low friction arthroplasty
LCM	left costal margin; lymphocytic choriomeningitis		
		LFC	living female child
		LFD	low fat diet; low forceps delivery; lactose free diet
LCR	late cutaneous reaction		
LCS	low constant suction; low continuous suction		
		LFP	left frontoposterior
L.C.T.	long chain triglyceride; low cervical transverse; lymphocytotoxicity	LFT	liver function tests; left frontotransverse; latex flocculation test
		lg	large; left gluteus
LCV	low cervical vertical	LGA	large for gestational age
LCX	left circumflex coronary artery	LGL	Lown-Ganong-Levine (syndrome)

LGV	lymphagranuloma venerum	LLB	long leg brace
LH	luteinizing hormone; left hyperphoria; left hand	LLC	long leg cast
		LLE	left lower extremity
LHF	left heart failure	LL-GXT	low-level graded exercise test
LHL	left hemisphere lesions	LLL	left lower lobe (lung); left lower lid
LHP	left hemiparesis		
LHR	leukocyte histamine release	LLO	Lengionella-like organism
LHRH	luteinizing hormone-releasing hormone (hypothalamic)	LLQ	left lower quadrant (abdomen)
		LLS	lazy leukocyte syndrome
LHT	left hypertropia	LLSB	left lower sternal border
Li	lithium		
LIB	left in bottle	LLT	left lateral thigh
LIC	left iliac crest; left internal carotid	LMA	left mento-anterior; liver membrane auto-antibody
LICA	left internal carotid artery		
		LMB	Laurence-Moon-Biedl syndrome
LiCO₃	lithium carbonate	LMC	living male child
LIF	left iliac fossa; liver (migration) inhibitory factor	LMCA	left main coronary artery
		LMD	local medical doctor; low molecular weight dextran
LIG	ligament		
LIH	left inguinal hernia		
LIMA	left internal mammary artery (graft)	LMEE	left middle ear exploration
L.I.P.	lymphocytic interstitial pneumonia	L/min	liters per minute
		LML	left medial lateral
LIQ	liquid; lower inner quadrant	LMM	lentigo maligna melanoma
LIS	low intermittent suction		
LISS	low ionic strength saline	LMP	last menstrual period; left mentotposterior
LK	left kidney	LMT	left mentotransverse
LKKS	liver, kidneys, spleen	LMWD	low molecular weight dextran
LKS	liver, kidneys, spleen		
LL	large lymphocyte; lumbar length; left leg; lower lip; lympho-blastic lymphoma	LN	lymph nodes
		LND	lymph node dissection
		LNMP	last normal menstrual period

LO	lateral oblique (x-ray view)	LRND	left radical neck dissection
LOA	left occiput anterior; leave of absence	LRQ	lower right quadrant
		L-S	lumbo-sacral
LOC	loss of consciousness; laxative of choice; level of consciousness; level of care; local	L/S	lecithin-spingo-myelin ratio
		LSA	left sacrum anterior; lipid-bound sialic acid; lymphosarcoma
LOD	line of duty		
LOL	little old lady	LSB	left sternal border
LOM	limitation of motion; left otitis media	LS BPS	laparoscopic bilateral partial salpingectomy
LoNa	low sodium	LSD	low salt diet; lysergide
LOP	leave on pass; left occiput posterior	LSE	local side effects
		LSF	low saturated fat
LOQ	lower outer quadrant	LSKM	liver-spleen-kidney-megalia
LORS-I	Level of Rehabilitation Scale-I		
		LSM	late systolic murmur
LOS	length of stay	LSO	left salpingo-oophorectomy
LOT	left occiput transverse		
LOV	loss of vision	LSP	left sacrum posterior; liver-specific (mem-brane) lipoprotein
LOZ	lozenge		
LP	lumbar puncture; light perception	L-Spar	Elspar (asparaginase)
L-PAM	melphalan	L/S ratio	lecithin/sphingomyelin ratio
LPC	laser photocoagulation		
lpf	low-power field	LSS	liver-spleen scan
LPD	luteal phase defect	LST	left sacrum transverse
LPH	left posterior hemiblock	L.S.T.L.	laparoscopic tubal ligation
LPN	licensed practical nurse	LT	light; left; lumbar trac-tion; left thigh; levin tube; leukotrienes
LPO	left posterior oblique; light perception only		
LPP	lipoprotein lipase	LTB	laparoscopic tubal banding; laryngo-tracheo-bronchitis
LPS	lipopolysaccharide		
LR	light reflex; labor room; left-right; lac-tated Ringer's (injection)	LTC	left to count; long-term care
		LTCF	long-term care facility
L→R	left to right	LTCS	low transverse cesarean section
LRD	living renal donor		

LTGA	left transposition of great artery	L & W	living and well
LTL	laparoscopic tubal ligation	LWCT	Lee-White clotting time
LTT	lymphocyte transformation test	LYG	lymphmatoid granulomatosis
L & U	lower and upper	lymphs	lymphocytes
LUE	left upper extremity	lytes	electrolytes (Na, K, Cl, etc.)
LUL	left upper lobe (lung)		
LUQ	left upper quadrant		
LUSB	left upper sternal border		

LV left ventricle

LVA left ventricular aneurysm

LVAD left ventricular assist device

LVE left ventricular enlargement

LVEDP left ventricular end diastolic pressure

LVEDV left ventricular end diastolic volume

LVEF left ventricular ejection fraction

LVF left ventricular failure

LVFP left ventricular filling pressure

LVH left ventricular hypertrophy

LVL left vastus lateralis

LVMM left ventricular muscle mass

LVP left ventricular pressure; large volume parenteral

LVPW left ventricular posterior wall

LVSWI left ventricular stroke work index

LVV left ventricular volume

M

M murmur; monocytes; male; molar; married; meter; minimum; medial; thousand; myopia

M_1 first mitral sound

M^2 square meters (body surface)

M.A. mental age; medical assistance; milliamps; Miller-Abbott (tube); menstrual age

M/A mood and/or affect

MAA macroaggregates of albumin

MAB monoclonal antibody

MABP mean arterial blood pressure

MAC maximal allowable concentration; mid-arm circumference; minimum alveolar concentration

MAE moves all extremities

MAEEW moves all extremities equally well

MAFAs movement-associated fetal (heart rate) accelerations

mag cit magnesium citrate

mag sulf magnesium sulfate

MAHA	macroangiopathic hemolytic anemia	MCA	middle cerebral aneurysm; middle cerebral artery; motorcycle accident; monoclonal antibodies
MAI	mycobacterium avium-intracellulare		
MAL	midaxillary line		
MALT	mucosa-associated lymphoid tissue	MCC	midstream clean-catch
MAMC	mid-arm muscle circumference	mcg (µg)	microgram
Mammo	mammography	MCGN	minimal-change glomerular nephritis
MAOI	monoamine oxidase inhibitor	MCH	mean corpuscular hemoglobin; muscle contraction headache
Mand	mandibular		
MAP	mean arterial pressure	MCHC	mean corpuscular hemoglobin concentration
MAS	meconium aspiration syndrome; mobile arm support		
		MCL	midclavicular line; midcostal line
MAST	military antishock trousers	MCLNS	mucocutaneous lymph node syndrome
MAT	multifocal atrial tachycardia	MCP	metacarpophalangeal joint
max	maximal; maxillary	MCS	microculture and sensitivity
M-BACOD	a drug combination protocol	MCSA	minimal cross-sectional area
MBC	maximum breathing capacity; minimal bacteriocidal concentration	MCT	medium chain triglyceride; mean circulation time
MB-CK	a creatinine kinase isoenzyme	MCTD	mixed connective tissue disease
MBD	minimal brain damage; minimal brain dysfunction	MCV	mean corpuscular volume
MBI	methylene blue installation	MD	medical doctor; mental deficiency; muscular dystrophy; manic depression
MBM	mothers breast milk		
MC	mixed cellularity; metatarso-cuneiform; monocomponent highly purified pork insulin	MDA	methylenedioxyamphetamine; manual dilation of the anus
		MDC	medial dorsal cutaneous (nerve)

MDD	manic depressive disorder; major depressive disorder	MEOS	microsomal ethanol oxidizing system
MDF	myocardial depressant factor	mEq	milliequivalent
MDI	multiple daily injection; metered dose inhaler	M/E ratio	myeloid/erythroid ratio
		META	metamyelocytes
		METHb	methemoglobin
MDII	multiple daily insulin injection	METS	metabolic equivalents (multiples of resting oxygen uptake)
MDM	middiastolic murmur; minor determinant mix (of penicillin)	MF	myocardial fibrosis; mycosis fungoides; midcavity forceps
MDP	methylene diphosphorate	M & F	mother and father; male and female
M.D.R.	minimum daily requirement	MFA	mid-forceps delivery
MDS	maternal deprivation syndrome	MFAT	multifocal atrial tachycardia
MDTP	multidisciplinary treatment plan	MFEM	maximal forced expiratory maneuver
ME	macula edema; medical examiner; middle ear	MFH	malignant fibrous histiocytoma
MEA-I	multiple endocrine adenomatosis type I	MFR	mid-forceps rotation
		MG	myasthenia gravis; milligram; Marcus Gunn
mec	meconium	Mg	magnesium
MeCCNU	semustine	MGBG	methyl-GAG (methylglyoxal bisguanylhydrazone)
MED	medical; medication; medicine; medium; median erythrocyte diameter; medial	MGF	maternal grandfather
MEDAC	multiple endocrine deficiency-autoimmune-candidiasis	MGM	maternal grandmother; milligram (mg is correct)
MEE	middle ear effusion	MgO	magnesium oxide
MEF	maximum expired flow rate	$MgSO_4$	magnesium sulfate
MEFV	maximum expiratory flow-volume	MGUS	monoclonal gammapathies of undetermined significance
MEL B	melarsoprol		
MEN (II)	multiple endocrine neoplasia (type II)	M-GXT	multi-stage graded exercise test

MH	marital history; menstrual history; mental health; malignant hyperthermia
MHA	microangiopathic hemolytic anemia
MHB	maximum hospital benefit; methemoglobin
MHC	major histocompatibility complex; mental health center
MH/MR	mental health & mental retardation
MI	myocardial infarction; mitral insufficiency; mental institution
MIA	medically indigent adult; missing in action
MIC	minimum inhibitory concentration; maternal and infant care
MICN	mobile intensive care nurse
MICU	medical intensive care unit; mobile intensive care unit
MIF	migration inhibitory factor; merthiolate-iodine-formalin
MIH	migraine with interparoxysmal headache
min	minimum; minute; minor
MIO	minimum identifiable odor
MIRP	myocardial infarction rehabilitation program
misc	miscellaneous
MISO	misonidazole
MITO-C	mitomycin
mix mon	mixed monitor
MJT	Mead Johnson tube

ML	midline; milliliter; middle lobe
mL	milliliter
MLC	mixed lymphocyte culture; minimal lethal concentration
MLD	metachromatic leukodystrophy; minimal lethal dose
MLF	median longitudinal fasciculus
MLNS	mucocutaneous lymph node syndrome
MLR	mixed lymphocyte reaction
MM	millimeter; mucous membrane; multiple myeloma
mM.	millimole
M&M	milk and molasses; morbidity and mortality
MMECT	multiple monitor electroconvulsive therapy
MMC	mitomycin (mitomycin C)
MMEFR	maximal midexpiratory flow rate
MMF	mean maximum flow
MMFR	maximal mid-expiratory flow rate
mmHg	millimeters of mercury
MMK	Marshall-Marchetti-Krantz (cystourethroplexy)
MMOA	maxillary mandibular odentectomy alveolectomy
mmol	millimole
MMPI	Minnesota Multiphasic Personality Inventory

MMR	measles, mumps, rubella; midline malignant reticulosis	mOsmol	milliosmole
MMS	Mini-Mental State (examination)	MP	metacarpal phalangeal joint; mercaptopurine
MMT	manual muscle test	6-MP	mercaptopurine
MMWR	Morbidity & Mortality Weekly Report	MPGN	membranoproliferative glomeruloephritis
MN	midnight	MPH	Master of Public Health; methyl-phenidate
Mn	manganese		
M&N	morning and night	MPJ	metacarpophalangeal joint
MNC	mononuclear leukocytes		
MNG	multinodular goiter	MPL	maximum permissable level
MNR	marrow neutrophil reserve	MPS	mucopolysaccharidosis
Mn SSEPS	median nerve somato-sensory evoked potentials	MPTR↓	motor, pain, touch, reflex deficit
		MR	mental retardation; may repeat; magnetic resonance; mitral regurgitation
MNTB	medial nucleus of the trapezoid body		
MO	mineral oil; month; medial oblique (x-ray view)	MR × 1	may repeat times one (once)
Mo	molybdenum	MRA	medical record administrator
MOA	mechanism of action		
MOB	medical office building	MRAN	medical resident admitting note
MOD	moderate; medical officer of the day	MRD	Medical Records Department
MODY	maturity onset diabetes of the youth	MRG	murmurs, rubs and gallops
MOF	methotrexate, Oncovin®, and fluorouracil; multiple organ failure	MRI	magnetic resonance imaging
		mRNA	messenger ribonucleic acid
MOM	milk of magnesia	MRS	methicillin resistant Staphylococcus aureus; magnetic resonance spectroscopy
mono.	monocyte; infectious mononucleosis		
MOPP	mechlorethamine, vicristine, procarba-zine, prednisone		
mOsm	milliosmole		

MS	morphine sulfate; multiple sclerosis; mitral stenosis; musculoskeletal; medical student; minimal support; muscle strength; mental status		MTM	modified Thayer-Martin medium
			MTP	metatarsal phalangeal
			MTU	methylthiouracil; malignant teratoma undifferentiated
M & S	microculture and sensitivity		MTX	methotrexate
			MU	million units
MSAF	meconium stained amniotic fluid		MUGA	multiple gated acquisition
MSAFP	maternal serum alpha fetoprotein		MUGX	multiple gated acquisition exercise
MSE	Mental Status Examination		MVA	motor vehicle accident; malignant vertricular arrhythmias
MSG	monosodium glutamate; methysergide		MVB	mixed venous blood
			MVC	maximal voluntary contraction
MSH	melanocyte-stimulating hormone		MVI®	trade name for parenteral multivitamins
MSK	medullary sponge kidney		MVI 12®	trade name for parenteral multivitamins
MSL	midsternal line			
MSO$_4$	morphine sulfate (this is a dangerous abbreviation)		MVO$_2$	myocardial oxygen consumption
			MVP	mitral valve prolapse
MSR	muscle stretch reflexes		MVR	mitral valve replacement; mitral valve regurgitation
MSS	minor surgery suite; muscular subaortic stenosis; Marital Satisfaction Scale			
			MVS	mitral valve stenosis
			MVV	maximum voluntary ventilation; mixed vespid venom
MST	mean survival time			
MSTA®	mumps skin test antigen		MWS	Mickety-Wilson syndrome
MSU	midstream urine			
MSUD	maple-syrup urine disease		My	myopia
			myelo	myelocytes
MSW	multiple stab wounds; Master of Social Work			
MT	music therapy; empty			

N

MTD	Monroe Tidal drainage
MTI	malignant teratoma intermiate

N	normal; negro; never; no; not; NPH insulin; negative

5'-N	5'-Nucleotidase	NBTE	nonbacterial thrombotic endocarditis
Na	sodium		
NA	nursing assistant; not applicable; nurse anesthetist	NC	neurologic check; no complaints; not completed; nasal cannula
NAA	neutron activation analysis	NCA	neurocirculatory asthenia
NABS	normoactive bowel sounds	NCAS	neocarzinostatin
NaCl	sodium chloride (salt)	NC/AT	normal cephalic atraumatic
NAD	no acute distress; no apparent distress; no appreciable disease; normal axis deviation; nothing abnormal detected	NCB	no code blue
		NCD	normal childhood diseases; not considered disabling
		NCF	neutrophilic chemotactic factor
NADPH	nicotinamide adenine dinucleotide phosphate	NCI	National Cancer Institute
NaF	sodium fluoride	NCJ	needle catheter jejunostomy
NAG	narrow angle glaucoma		
$NaHCO_3$	sodium bicarbonate	NCL	neuronal ceroid lipofuscinosis
NaI	sodium iodide		
NANB	non-A, non-B (hepatitis)	NCM	nailfold capillary microscope
NAPA	N-acetyl procainamide	NCNC	normochromic, normocytic
Na Pent	Pentothal Sodium®	NCPR	no cardiopulmonary resuscitation
NAS	no added salt; neonatal abstinence syndrome	NCS	zinostatis (neocarzinostatin); no concentrated sweets; nerve conduction studies
NAT	no action taken		
NB	newborn; note well; needle biopsy		
		NCV	nerve conduction velocity
NBM	nothing by mouth; no bowel movement; normal bowel movement	ND	normal delivery; normal development; not done; nasal deformity; not diagnosed
NBN	newborn nursery		
NBS	normal bowel sound; no bacteria seen	Nd	neodymium
		NDA	new drug application
NBT	nitroblue tetrazolium reduction (tests)	NDD	no dialysis days

NDT	neurodevelopmental treatment	NICU	neurosurgical intensive care unit; neonatal intensive care unit
NDV	Newcastle disease virus		
NE	norepinephrine; not elevated; not examined	NIDD	non-insulin-dependent diabetes
NEC	necrotizing enterocolitis; not elsewhere classified	NIDDM	non-insulin-dependent diabetes mellitus
		NIF	negative inspiratory force
NED	no evidence of disease		
NEG	negative	NIH	National Institutes of Health
NEMD	nonspecific esophageal motility disorder	NINVS	non-invasive neurovascular studies
NET	naso-endotracheal tube		
NF	negro female; not found; neurofibromatosis	Nitro	nitroglycerin; sodium nitroprusside
		NJ	nasojejunal
NFL	nerve fiber layer	NK	natural killer (cells)
NFTD	normal full term delivery	NKA	no known allergies
		NKDA	no known drug allergies
NFTT	nonorganic failure to thrive	NKHS	nonketotic hyperosmolar syndrome
NFW	nursed fairly well	NKMA	no known medication allergies
NG	nasogastric; nanogram; nitroglycerin		
		NL	normal
n giv	not given	NLD	necrobiosis lipoidica diabeticorum; nasolacrimal duct
NGR	nasogastric replacement		
NGT	nasogastric tube		
NGU	nongonococcal urethritis	NLF	nasolabial fold
		NLP	nodular liquifying panniculitis; no light perception
NH	nursing home		
NH$_4$Cl	ammonium chloride		
NHD	normal hair distribution	NLT	not later than; not less than
NHL	non-Hodgkin's lymphomas; nodular histiocytic lymphoma	NM	negro male; neuromuscular; nodular melanoma
NHP	nursing home placement		
		NMD	normal muscle development
NICC	neonatal intensive care center		

NMR	nuclear magnetic resonance (same as magnetic resonance imaging)	NPC	near point convergences; nodal premature contractions; nonpatient contact
NMI	no middle initial	NPDL	nodular poorly differentiated lymphocytic
NMS	neuroleptic malignant syndrome	NPDR	nonproliferative diabetic retinopathy
NMT	no more than	NPH	normal pressure hydrocephalus; a type of insulin (Isophane); no previous history
NN	neonatal; nurses' notes		
NND	neonatal death		
NNE	neonatal necrotizing enterocolitis		
NNM	Nicolle-Novy-MacNeal (media)	NPhx	nasopharynx
NNO	no new orders	NPI	no present illness
		NPN	nonprotein nitrogen
NNP	neonatal nurse practitioner	NPO	nothing by mouth
NNU	net nitrogen utilization	NPT	normal pressure and temperature; nocturnal penile tumescence
no.	number		
N$_2$O	nitrous oxide	NR	nonreactive
N$_2$O:O$_2$	nitrous oxide to oxygen ratio	NRBS	non-rebreathing system
noc.	night	NRC	normal retinal correspondence
noct	nocturnal		
NOD	notify of death	NREM	nonrapid eye movement
NOMI	nonocclusive mesenteric infarction	NREMS	nonrapid eye movement sleep
NOOB	not out of bed	NRT	neuromuscular reeducation techniques
NOR	nortriptyline		
NOR-EPI	norepinephrine	NS	normal saline solution (0.9% sodium chloride solution); nephrotic syndrome; nuclear sclerosis; not seen; nylon suture; not significant
NOS	not otherwise specified		
NOSIE	Nurse Observation Scale for Inpatient Evaluation		
NP	neuropsychiatric; nasopharyngeal; newly presented; no pain; not pregnant; not present; nursed poorly; nasal prongs; neurophysin		
		NSA	normal serum albumin; no significant abnormality
		NSABP	National Surgical Adjuvant Breast Project
NPA	near point of accommodation	NSAIA	non-steroidal anti-inflammatory agent

NSAID	non-steroidal anti-inflammatory drug		NSVD	normal spontaneous vaginal delivery
NSC	no significant change; not service connected		NT	not tested; naso-tracheal; not tender
NSCLC	non-small-cell lung cancer		N&T	nose and throat
NSD	normal spontaneous delivery; nominal standard dose		NTC	neurotrauma center
			NTE	not to exceed
			NTF	normal throat flora
NSDA	non-steroid dependent asthmatic		NTG	nitroglycerin; non-treatment group
NSE	neuron-specific enolase		NTMB	nontuberculous myo-bacteria
NSFTD	normal spontaneous full-term delivery		NTMI	non-transmural myocardial infarction
NSG	nursing		NTP	Nitropaste® (nitro-glycerin ointment); sodium nitroprusside; normal temperature and pressure
NSILA	nonsuppressible insulin-like activity			
NSN	nephrotoxic serum nephritis			
NSO	Neosporin® ointment		NTS	nasotracheal suction; nucleus tractus solitarii
NSPVT	nonsustained poly-morphic ventricular tachycardia			
			NTT	nasotracheal tube
NSR	normal sinus rhythm; not seen regularly; nonspecific reaction; nasoseptal repair		NUD	nonulcer dyspepsia
			nullip	nullipara
			NV	neurovascular
			N&V	nausea and vomiting
NSS	sodium chloride 0.9% (normal saline solution)		NVD	neck vein distention; nausea, vomiting, and diarrhea; no venereal disease; neurovesicle dysfunction; nonvalvu-lar disease; neovascu-larization of the disc
1/2 NSS	sodium chloride 0.45% (1/2 normal saline solution)			
NSSTT	nonspecific ST and T (wave)			
			NVE	neovascularization elsewhere
NST	nutritional support team; non-stress test; not sooner than		NVG	neovascular glaucoma
			NVS	neurological vital signs
NSU	nonspecific urethritis		NWB	non-weight bearing
NSV	nonspecific vaginitis		NYD	not yet diagnosed

O

O	oxygen; objective findings; eye; oral; open; obvious; often; other; occlusal
ō	negative; without; none
$_1O_2$	singlet oxygen
O_2	oxygen; both eyes
O_{2v}	superoxide
OA	oral alimentation; Overeaters Anonymous; occiput anterior; osteoarthritis
O & A	observation & assessment
OAF	osteoclast activating factor
Ob	obstetrics
OB	occult blood
OBE-CALP	placebo capsule or tablet
Ob-Gyn	obstetrics and gynecology
OBS	organic brain syndrome
OC	oral contraceptive; obstetrical conjugate; oral care; on call; office call
OCA	oculocutaneous albinism
OCCC	open chest cardiac compression
OCCM	open chest cardiac massage
OCG	oral cholecystogram
OCP	ova, cysts, parasites
OCT	ornithine carbamyl transferase; oxytocin challenge test
OCU	observation care unit
OD	right eye; overdose; on duty; doctor of optometry (also a dangerous abbreviation for once daily)
Δ OD 450	deviation of optical density at 450
OER	oxygen enhancement ratios
OFC	occipital-frontal circumference
OG	orogastric (feeding)
OGTT	oral glucose tolerance test
OH	occupational history; open heart
17 OH	17-hydroxycortico-steroids
OHA	oral hypoglycemic agents
OH Cbl	hydroxycobalamine
OHD	organic heart disease; hydroxy vitamin D
OHF	omsk hemorrhagic fever
OHG	oral hypoglycemic
OHIAA	hydroxyindolacetic acid
OHP	oxygen under hyperbaric pressure
OHRR	open heart recovery room
OHS	open heart surgery
OI	osteogenesis imperfecta
OIF	oil-immersion field
OJ	orthoplast jacket; orange juice (this is a dangerous abbreviation)
OKAN	optokinetic after nystagmus
OKN	optokinetic nystagmus

OLA	occiput left anterior	OPS	operations
OM	otitis media; every morning (this is a dangerous abbreviation)	OPV	oral polio vaccine
		OR	operating room; oil retention
OME	office of Medical Examiner; otitis media with effusion	ORIF	open reduction internal fixation
		ORL	otorhinolaryngology
OMI	old myocardial infarct	OS	left eye; opening snap; mouth (this is a dangerous abbreviation); osmium
OMR	operative mortality rate		
OMSC	otitis media secretory (or suppurative) chronic		
		OSA	obstructive sleep apnea
ON	overnight; Ortho-Novum®; every night (this is a dangerous abbreviation)	OSD	overside drainage
		OSM S	osmolarity serum
		OSM U	osmolarity urine
		OSN	off service note
ONC	over-the-needle catheter	OSS	osseous
		OT	old tuberculin; occupational therapy
OOB	out of bed		
OOBBRP	out of bed with bathroom privileges	OTC	over the counter (sold without prescription)
OOC	out of control	OTD	out the door
OOP	out on pass; out of pelvis	OTH	other
		OTO	otology
OOR	out of room	OTR	Occupational Therapist, Registered
OOT	out of town		
OP	outpatient; operation; occiput posterior; open	OTS	orotracheal suction
		OTT	orotracheal tube
O&P	ova and parasites	OU	both eyes
OPB	outpatient basis	OV	office visit; ovum; ovary
OPC	outpatient clinic		
OPCA	olivopontocerebellar atrophy	OW	out of wedlock
		oz	ounce
OPD	outpatient department		
O'p'-DDD	mitotane		

P

OPG	ocular plethysmography
OPM	occult primary malignancy
OPPG	oculopneumoplethysmography

P	plan; protein; pint; pulse; peripheral; phosphorous; para
p	after

P_2	pulmonic second heart sound
^{32}P	radioactive phosphorous
PA	posterior-anterior (x-ray); pulmonary artery; pernicious anemia; physician assistant; presents again; psychiatric aide; professional association; phenol alcohol
P&A	percussion and auscultation
PAB	premature atrial beat
PAC	premature atrial contraction
PACH	pipers to after coming head
PADP	pulmonary artery diastolic pressure
PAF	paroxysmal atrial fibrillation; platelet activating factors
PAO₂	arterial oxygen tension
PaCO₂	arterial carbon dioxide tension
PAGE	polyacrylamide gel electrophoresis
PAH	para-aminohippurate
PAIVS	pulmonary atresia with intact ventricle septum
Pa Line	pulmonary artery line
PALN	para-aortic lymph node
PAM	penicillin aluminum monostearate
PAN	periodic alternating nystagmus; polyarteritis nodosa
PAOP	pulmonary artery occlusion pressure

PAP	pulmonary artery pressure; prostatic acid phosphatase
Pap smear	Papanicolaou smear
PA/PS	pulmonary atresia/pulmonary stenosis
PAR	postanesthetic recovery; platelet aggregate ratio
PARA para	number of pregnancies paraplegic
PARU	postanesthetic recovery unit
PAS	periodic acid-Schiff (reagent); peripheral anterior synechia; pulmonary artery stenosis
PAS or PASA	para-aminosalicyclic acid
Pas Ex	passive exercise
PAT	paroxysmal atrial tachycardia; preadmission testing; percent acceleration time
Path.	pathology
PAWP	pulmonary artery wedge pressure
Pb	lead; phenobarbital
PB	powder board; parafin bath
P&B	phenobarbital & belladonna
PBA	percutaneous bladder aspiration
PBC	point of basal convergence; primary biliary cirrhosis
PBD	percutaneous biliary drainage
PBG	porphobilinogen

PBI	protein-bound iodine	PCO	polycystic ovary
PBL	peripheral blood lymphocyte	PCO$_2$	carbon dioxide pressure (or tension)
PBMC	peripheral blood mononuclear cell	PCOD	polycystic ovarian disease
PBMNC	peripheral blood mononuclear cell	PCP	phencyclidine; pneumonocystis carinii pneumonia; pulmonary capillary pressure
PBN	polymyxin B sulfate, bacitracin and neomycin		
		PCR	protein catabolic rate
PBO	placebo	PCT	porphyria cutanea tarda; post coital test
PBZ	pyribenzamine; phenylbutazone; phenoxybenzamine		
		PCV	packed cell volume
ΦBZ	phenylbutazone	PCWP	pulmonary capillary wedge pressure
PC	after meal; packed cells; professional corporation; platelet concentrate	PCZ	prochlorperazine; procarbazine
		PD	peritoneal dialysis; postural drainage; Parkinson's disease; interpupillary distance; percutaneous drain
PCA	patient care assistant (aide); patient controlled analgesia; posterior cerebral artery; procoagulation activity; passive cutaneous anaphylaxis		
		P/D	packs per day (cigarettes)
		PDA	patent ductus arteriosus
PCB	pancuronium bromide	PDD	cisplatin
PCCU	post coronary care unit	PDE	paroxysmal dyspnea on exertion; pulsed Doppler echocardiography
PCG	phonocardiogram		
PCH	paroxysmal cold hemoglobinuria		
PCI	prophylactic cranial irradiation	PDFC	premature dead female child
PCIOL	posterior chamber intraocular lens	PDGF	platelet derived growth factor
PCL	posterior chamber lens; posterior cruciate ligament	PDL	poorly differentiated lymphocytic
		PDL-D	poorly differentiated lymphocytic-diffuse
PCM	protein-calorie malnutrition	PDL-N	poorly differentiated lymphocytic-nodular
PCMX	chloroxylenol		
PCN	penicillin		

PDMC	premature dead male child	perf.	perforation
PDN	prednisone; private duty nurse	PERL	pupils equal, reactive to light
PDR	proliferative diabetic retinopathy; Physician's Desk Reference	per os	by mouth (this is a dangerous abbreviation)
PDS	pain dysfunction syndrome	PERR	pattern evoked retinal response
PDGXT	predischarge graded exercise test	PERRLA	pupils, equal, round, reactive to light and accommodation
PDT	photodynamic therapy	PES	pre-excitation syndrome
PDU	pulsed Doppler ultrasonography	PET	positron-emission tomography; pre-eclamptic toxemia; pressure equalizing tubes
PE	physical examination; pulmonary embolism; pressure equalization; plural effusion; polyethylene		
		PETN	pentaerythritol tetranitrate
P_1E_1®	epinephrine 1%, pilocarpine 1% ophthalmic solution	PEx	physical examination
		PF	power factor
PECHO	prostatic echogram	PFC	persistent fetal circulation
$PECO_2$	mixed expired carbon dioxide tension	PFM	porcelain fused to metal
Peds.	pediatrics	PFR	peak flow rate; parotid flow rate
PEEP	positive end-expiratory pressure		
PEFR	peak expiratory flow rate	PFT	pulmonary function test
PEG	pneumoencephalogram; polyethylene glycol; percutaneous endoscopic gastrostomy	PFU	plaque-forming unit
		PG	pregnant; paregoric; polygalacturonate; phosphatidyl glycerol
PEN	parenteral and enteral nutrition		
		PGA	prostaglandin
PENS	percutaneous epidural nerve stimulator	PGE2	prostaglandin E2
		PGF	paternal grandfather
PEP	protein electrophoresis; pre-ejection period	PGF2 α	prostaglandin F2 α
		PGH	pituitary growth hormones
PER	pediatric emergency room	PGL	persistent generalized lymphadenopathy

PGM	paternal grandmother	PIE	pulmonary infiltration with eosinophilia; pulmonary interstitial emphysema
PgR	progesterone receptor		
PGU	postgonococcal urethritis		
*p*H	hydrogen ion concentration	PIH	pregnancy induced hypertension
PH	past history; poor health; public health	PISA	phase invariant signature algorithm
Ph¹	Philadelphia chromosome	PIO	pemoline
		PIOK	poikilocytosis
PHA	passive hemagglutinating; phytohemagglutinin; arterial pH; phytohemagglutinin antigen	PIP	proximal interphalangeal joint; post inspiratory pressure
		Pit	Pitocin®; Pitressin® (this is a dangerous abbreviation)
Pharm	Pharmacy		
PHC	primary hepatocellular carcinoma	PITR	plasma iron turnover rate
PHH	posthemorrhagic hydrocephalus	PIV	peripheral intravenous
		PIVD	protruded intervertebral disc
PHN	public health nurse; post herpetic neuralgia	PJB	premature junctional beat
PHPT	primary hyperparathyroidism	PJC	premature junctional contractions
PHPV	persistent hyperplastic primary vitreous	PJS	Peutz-Jeghers syndrome
PHx	past history	PK	penetrating keratoplasty
Phx	pharynx		
PI	present illness; pulmonary infarction; peripheral iridectomy	PKD	polycystic kidney disease
		PK Test	Prausnitz-Kunstner transfer test
PIAT	Peabody Individual Achievement Test	PKU	phenylketonuria
PICA	posterior inferior communicating artery; posterior inferior cerebellar artery	PL	plantar; place; light perception
		PLAP	placental alkaline phosphatase
PICU	pediatric intensive care unit	PLFC	premature living female child
PID	pelvic inflammatory disease; prolapsed intervertebral disc	PLH	paroxysmal localized hyperhidrosis

PLL	prolymphocytic leukemia	PMTS	premenstrual tension syndrome
PLMC	premature living male child	PMV	prolapse of mitral valve
PLN	pelvic lymph node; popliteal lymph node	PMW	pacemaker wires
		PN	parenteral nutrition; progress note; percussion note
PLS	primary lateral sclerosis		
plts	platelets	PNAS	prudent no salt added
PM	post mortem, evening; pretibial myxedema; presents mainly; primary motivation	PNB	premature nodal beat
		PNC	premature nodal contraction; peripheral nerve conduction
PMA	Prinzmetal's angina; premenstrual asthma	PND	paroxysmal nocturnal dyspnea; postnasal drip
PMB	postmenopausal bleeding; polymorphonuclear basophil (leukocytes)	PNET-MB	primitive neuro-ectodermal tumors-medulloblastoma
PMC	pseudomembranous colitis	PNF	proprioceptive neuro-muscular fasciculation reaction
PMD	private medical doctor		
PME	post menopausal estrogen	PNH	paroxysmal nocturnal hemoglobinuria
PMF	progressive massive fibrosis	PNI	prognostic nutrition index; peripheral nerve injury
PMH	past medical history		
PMI	point of maximal impulse; patient medication instructions	PNMG	persistent neonatal myasthenia gravis
PMN	polymorphonuclear leukocyte	PNP	Pediatric Nurse Practitioner; progressive nuclear palsey
PMP	previous menstrual period; pain management program	PNS	peripheral nervous system; partial nonprogressing stroke; practical nursing student
PMR	polymyalgia rheumatica; polymorphic reticulosis		
PM&R	physical medicine and rehabilitation	PNT	percutaneous nephrostomy tube
PMS	postmenstrual syndrome	PNU	protein nitrogen units
		PNV	prenatal vitamins
PMT	premenstrual tension	Pnx	pneumothorax

PO	by mouth (per os); phone order; post-operative	PP	postpartum; post-prandial; paradoxical pulse; pin prick; pro-toporphyria; proximal phalanx; private patient; near point of accommodation
PO_2	partial pressure of oxygen		
PO_4	phosphate		
POA	pancreatic oncofetal antigen	P&P	pins and plaster
POAG	primary open-angle glaucoma	PPA	phenylpropanolamine
		PPB	parts per billion
POC	product of conception; postoperative care	PPBS	post prandial blood sugar
POD 1	postoperative day one	PPC	progressive patient care
POEMS	plasma cell dyscasia with polyneuropathy, organomegaly, endo-crinopathy, mono-clonal (M)-protein, skin changes	PPD	purified protein deriva-tive (of tuberculin); packs per day; post-partum day; posterior polymorphous dys-trophy
POIK	poikilocytosis	P & PD	percussion & postural drainage
POL	premature onset of labor	PPD-B	purified protein deriva-tive, Battey
POLY	polymorphonuclear leukocyte	PPD-S	purified protein deriva-tive, standard
POMP	prednisone, vincristine, methotrexate, mercap-topurine	PPF	plasma protein fraction
		PPG	photoplethysmography
POMR	problem-oriented med-ical record	PPH	postpartum hemor-rhage
POp	postoperative	PPHN	persistent pulmonary hypertension of the newborn
poplit	popliteal		
POR	problem-oriented record	PPI	patient package insert
PORP	partial ossicular replacement prosthesis	PPL	pars planus lensectomy
		PPLO	pleuro-pneumonia-like organisms
PORT	postoperative respira-tory therapy	PPM	parts per million
POS	parosteal osteosarcoma	PPN	peripheral parenteral nutrition
poss	possible		
post	post mortem examina-tion (autopsy)	PPNG	penicillinase producing Neisseria gonorrhoeae
post op	postoperative		

PPO	prefered provider organization	PROM	passive range of motion; premature rupture of membranes
PPP	postpartum psychosis		
PPPG	post prandial plasma glucose	ProMACE	a drug combination protocol
PPPBL	peripheral pulses palpable both legs	prov	provisional
PPROM	prolonged premature rupture of membranes	PRP	polyribose ribitol phosphate; panretinal photocoagulation
PPS	postpartum sterilization		
PPTL	postpartum tubal ligation	PRPP	5-phosphoribosyl-1-pyrophosphate
PPVT	Peabody Picture Vocabulary Test	PRRE	pupils round regular, equal
PR	Puerto Rican; per rectum; pulse rate; profile; far point of accommodation	PRSs	positive rolandic spikes
		PRTH-C	prothrombin time control
P & R	pulse and respiration; pelvic & rectal	PRV	polycythemia rubra vera
PRA	plasma renin activity	PRVEP	pattern reversal visual evoked potentials
PRAT	platelet radioactive antiglobulin test		
PRBC	packed red blood cells	PRW	polymerized ragweed
PRCA	pure red cell aplasia	PRZF	pyrazofurin
PRE	progressive resistive exercise	PS	pulmonary stenosis; paradoxic sleep; pathologic stage; plastic surgery; serum from pregnant women; performance status
Pred	prednisone		
pre-op	before surgery		
prep	prepare for surgery		
PRG	phleborrheogram		
PRIMP	primipara (1st pregnancy)	P & S	paracentesis and suction; pain and suffering
PRL	prolactin		
PRM-SDX	pyrimethamine sulfadoxine	PsA	psoriatic arthritis
PRN	as occasion requires	PS I	healthy patient with localized pathological process
PRO	protein		
prob	probable		
PROC-TO	procotoscopic; proctology	PS II	a patient with mild to moderate systemic disease
prog.	prognosis; prognathism		

74

PS III	a patient with severe systemic disease limiting activity but not incapacitating		PSW	psychiatric social worker
PS IV	a patient with incapacitating systemic disease		PSVT	paroxysmal supraventricular tachycardia
PS V	Moribund patient not expected to live.		PT	physical therapy; patient; prothrombin time; pine tar; posterior tibial; pint; phenytoin

(These are American Society of Anesthesiologists' physical status patient classifications. Emergency operations are designated by "E" after the classification).

PsA	psoriatic arthritis
PSC	posterior subcapsular cataract; primary sclerosing cholangitis
PSE	portal systemic encephalopathy
PSF	posterior spinal fusion
PSGN	post streptococcal glomerulonephritis
PSH	post spinal headache
PSI	pounds per square inch
PSM	presystolic murmur
PSP	phenolsulphthalein; pancreatic spasmolytic peptide; progressive supranuclear palsy
PSRBOW	premature spontaneous rupture of bag of waters
PSS	progressive systemic sclerosis; physiologic saline solution (0.9% sodium chloride)

PTA	prior to admission; plasma thromboplastin antecedent; pretreatment anxiety; pure-tone average; physical therapy assistant; percutaneous transluminal angioplasty
PTB	patellar tendon bearing
PTBD-EF	percutaneous transhepatic biliary drainage—enteric feeding
PTC	plasma thromboplastin components; percutaneous transhepatic cholangiography
PTCA	percutaneous transluminal coronary angioplasty
PTD	period to discharge; permanent and total disability
PTE	proximal tibial epiphysis; pulmonary thromboembolism; pretibial edema
PTFE	polytetrafluoroethylene
PTG	teniposide
PTH	post transfusion hepatitis; parathyroid hormone

PTL	pre-term labor; Sodium Pentothal®	PVD	patient very disturbed; peripheral vascular disease; posterior vitreous detachment
PTMDF	pupils, tension, media, disc, fundus		
pTNM	postsurgical resection-pathologic staging of cancer	PVE	premature ventricular extrasystole; perivenous encephalomyelitis
PTPM	posttraumatic progressive myelopathy	PVK	penicillin V potassium
PTPN	peripheral (vein) total parenteral nutrition	PVO	peripheral vascular occlusion; pulmonary venous occlusion
PTS	prior to surgery		
PTSD	post-traumatic stress disorder	PVOD	pulmonary vascular obstructive disease
PTT	partial thromboplastin time	PVP	peripheral venous pressure; polyvinyl-pyrrolidone
PTU	propylthiouracil		
PTX	pneumothorax	PVR	postvoiding residual; proliferative vitreoretinopathy; peripheral vascular resistance; pulse-volume recording
PU	peptic ulcer; pregnancy urine		
PUD	peptic ulcer disease		
PUFA	polyunsaturated fatty acids	PVS	peritoneovenous shunt; pulmonic valve stenosis; percussion, vibration and suction
pul.	pulmonary		
PUN	plasma urea nitrogen		
PUO	pyrexia of unknown origin	PVT	private
PUVA	psoralen-ultraviolet-light (treatment)	PWB	partial weight bearing
		PWLV	posterior wall of left ventricle
PV	polycythemia vera; polio vaccine; portal vein; pulmonary vein; per vagina	PWM	pokeweed mitogens
		PWP	pulmonary wedge pressure
P&V	pyloroplasty and vagotomy	PWV	polistes wasp venom
		Px	physical exam; pneumothorax; prognosis
PVA	polyvinyl alcohol		
PVB	premature ventricular beat	PXE	pseudoxanthoma elasticum
PVC	premature ventricular contraction; pulmonary venous congestion; polyvinyl chloride	PTx	parathyroidectomy
		PY	pack years
		PZA	pyrazinamide
		PZI	protamine zinc insulin

Q

q	every
QA	quality assurance
QAM	every morning (this is a dangerous abbreviation)
QCA	quantitative coronary angiography
qd	every day (this is a dangerous abbreviation)
q4h	every four hours
qh	every hour
qhs	every night (this is a dangerous abbreviation)
qid	four times daily
q.n.	every night (this is a dangerous abbreviation)
q.n.s.	quantity not sufficient
qod	every other day (this is a dangerous abbreviation)
qoh	every other hour (this is a dangerous abbreviation)
QON	every other night (this is a dangerous abbreviation)
qpm	every evening (this is a dangerous abbreviation)
QRS	principal deflection in an electrocardiogram
Q.S.	sufficient quantity; every shift
qt	quart
quad	quadriplegic
QUART	quadrantectomy, axillary dissection and radiotherapy
qwk	once a week (this is a dangerous abbreviation)

R

R	respiration; right; rectum; regular; rate; regular insulin
RA	rheumatoid arthritis; right atrium; right auricle; room air; right arm
RAA	renin-angiotensin-aldosterone
RABG	room air blood gas
RAC	right atrial catheter
RAD	radical; right axis deviation
RAE	right atrial enlargement
RAEB	refractory anemia, erythroblastic
RAG	room air gas
RAIU	radioactive iodine uptake
RALT	routine admission laboratory tests
RAM	rapid alternating movements
RAN	resident's admission notes
RAO	right anterior oblique
RAP	right atrial pressure
RAPD	relative afferent pupillary defect
RAS	renal artery stenosis
RAST	radioallergosorbent test
RAT	right anterior thigh

RA test	test for rheumatoid factor	RDH	Registered Dental Hygienist
R(AW)	airway resistance	RDS	respiratory distress syndrome
RB	retrobulbar; right buttock	RDT	regular dialysis (hemodialysis) treatment
R & B	right and below		
RBA	right brachial artery	RDVT	recurrent deep vein thrombosis
RBB	right breast biopsy		
RBBB	right bundle branch block	RE	reticuloendothelial; rectal examination; regional enteritis; concerning; right eye
RBCD	right border cardiac dullness		
RBC	red blood cell (count)		
RBD	right border of dullness	REE	resting energy expenditure
RBE	relative biologic effectiveness	REF	referred; renal erythropoietic factor
RBF	renal blood flow		
RBOW	rupture bag of water	rehab	rehabilitation
RBP	retinol-binding protein	Rel	religion
RBV	right brachial vein	REM	rapid eye movement
R/C	reclining chair	REMS	rapid eye movement sleep
RCA	right coronary artery; radionuclide cerebral angiogram	REP	repeat; report; repair
		repol	repolarization
RCC	renal cell carcinoma	RER	renal excretion rate
RCD	relative cardiac dullness	RES	reticuloendothelial system; resident
RCM	right costal margin; radiographic contrast media	RESC	resuscitation
		resp.	respiratory; respirations
RCS	reticulum cell sarcoma	retic	reticulocyte
RCT	root canal therapy	REV	revolutions; review; reverse
RCV	red cell volume		
R.D.	registered dietitian	RF	rheumatoid factor; renal failure; rheumatic fever
RD	renal disease; retinal detachment; respiratory disease		
		RFA	right fronto-anterior; right femoral artery
R.D.A.	recommended daily allowance	RFL	right frontolateral
		RFP	right frontoposterior
RDPE	reticular degeneration of the pigment epithelium	RFT	right frontotransverse
		RG	right gluteal

78

RGM	right gluteus medius	RL	right leg; right lung; right lateral; Ringer's lactate
Rh	Rhesus factor in blood		
RH	room humidifier; right hyperphoria; right hand; reduced halo-peridol	R→L	right to left
		RLE	right lower extremity
		RLF	retrolental fibroplasia
RHB	raise head of bed	RLL	right lower lobe
RHC	respiration has ceased	RLQ	right lower quadrant
RHD	rheumatic heart dis-ease; relative hepatic dullness	RLR	right lateral rectus
		RLT	right lateral thigh
		RM	repetitions maximum; room; radial mastec-tomy; respiratory movement
RHF	right heart failure		
RHL	right hemisphere lesions		
		R&M	routine and microscopic
RHT	right hypertropia	RMA	right mento-anterior
RI	regular insulin	RMCA	right main coronary artery
RIA	radioimmunoassay		
RIC	right iliac crest; right internal carotid (artery)	RMCL	right midclavicular line
		RMD	rapid movement disorder
RICS	right intercostal space		
RICU	respiratory intensive care unit	RME	right mediolateral episiotomy
		RMEE	right middle ear exploration
RID	radial immunodiffusion		
RIF	rifampin; rigid internal fixation; right iliac fossa	RML	right middle lobe
		RMP	right mentoposterior
		RMR	right medial rectus; resting metabolic rate
RIG	rabies immune globulin		
RIH	right inguinal hernia	RMS®	Rectal Morphine Sul-fate (suppository)
RIMA	right internal mammary anastamosis		
		RMSF	Rocky Mountain spotted fever
RIND	reversible ischemic neurologic defect		
		RMT	registered music thera-pist; right mentotrans-verse
RIP	radioimmunoprecipitin test; rapid infusion pump		
		RN	registered nurse
RISA	radioactive iodinated serum albumin	RNA	ribonucleic acid; radio-nuclide angiography
RIST	radioimmunosorbent test	RNEF	resting (radio-) nuclide ejection fraction
RK	radial keratotomy		

RND	radial neck dissection	RPLND	retroperitoneal lymphadenectomy
RO	routine order		
R/O	rule out	RPN	renal papillary necrosis
ROA	right occiput anterior	RPO	right posterior oblique
ROM	range of motion	RPP	rate-pressure product
ROP	right occiput posterior; retinopathy of prematurity	RPR	rapid plasma reagin (test for syphilis); Reiter protein reagin
ROS	review of systems		
ROSC	restoration of spontaneous circulation	RPT	Registered Physical Therapist
		RQ	respiratory quotient
RoRx	radiation therapy	RR	recovery room; respiratory rate; regular respirations
ROT	right occipital transverse; remedial occupational therapy		
		R&R	rate and rhythm
RQ	respiratory quotient	RRE	round, regular, and equal (pupils)
RP	retinitis pigmentosa; retrograde pyelogram; Raynaud's phenomenon		
		RREF	resting radionuclide ejection fraction
		rRNA	ribosomal ribonucleic acid
RPA	radial photon absorptiometry; right pulmonary artery		
		RRND	right radical neck dissection
RPCF	Reiter protein complement fixation	RRR	regular rhythm and rate
RPD	removable partial denture	RRRN	round, regular, react normally
RPE	retinal pigment epithelium; rating of perceived exertion	RS	rhythm strip; right side; Ringer's solution; Reiter's syndrome; Reye's syndrome
RPF	renal plasma flow; relaxed pelvic floor		
		RSA	right sacrum anterior; right subclavian artery
RPGN	rapidly progressive glomerulonephritis		
		RSDS	reflex-sympathetic dystrophy syndrome
RPH	retroperitoneal hemorrhage; Registered Pharmacist		
		R-SICU	respiratory-surgical intensive care unit
RPHA	reverse passive hemagglutination	RSO	right salpingo-oophorectomy
RPICCE	round pupil intracapsular cataract extraction	RSP	right sacroposterior
		RSR	regular sinus rhythm; relative survival rate

RSTs	Rodney Smith tubes	RVD	relative vertebral density
RSV	respiratory syncytial virus	RVE	right ventricular enlargement
RSW	right-sided weakness	RVET	right ventricular ejection time
RT	right; radiation therapy; recreational therapy; Respiratory Therapist; renal transplant; running total	RVG	radionuclide ventriculography
		RVH	right ventricular hypertrophy
R/t	related to	RVL	right vastus lateralis
RTA	renal tubular acidosis	RVO	retinal vein occlusion; relaxed vaginal outlet
RTC	return to clinic; round the clock	RVOT	right ventricular outflow tract
RTL	reactive to light	RVR	rapid ventricular response
RTM	routine medical care	RVSWI	right ventricular stroke work index
rTNM	retreatment staging of cancer	RV/TLC	residual volume to total lung capacity ratio
RTO	return to office		
RTOG	Radiation Therapy Oncology Group	RVV	rubella vaccine virus
rtPA	recombinant tissue-type plasminogen	Rx	therapy; drug; medication; treatment; take
RTRR	return to recovery room	RXN	reaction
RTS	real time scan		
RT$_3$U	resin triiodothyronine uptake		

S

RTx	radiation therapy	S	subjective findings; semilente insulin; serum; sister; single; suction; sacral
RUA	routine urine analysis		
RUE	right upper extremity		
RUG	retrograde urethrogram		
RUL	right upper lobe		
rupt.	ruptured	$\bar{s}$	without
RUQ	right upper quadrant	S$_1$	first heart sound; sacral vertebrae 1
RURTI	recurrent upper respiratory tract infection	S$_2$	second heart sound
RUSB	right upper sternal border	SA	sinoatrial; Spanish American; salicylic acid; sustained action; surface area; sinoatrial
RV	right ventricle; residual volume; rectovaginal; rubella vaccine		

S/A	sugar and acetone	SBGM	self blood glucose monitoring
SAB	subarachnoid block; subarachnoid bleed	SBI	systemic bacterial infection
SAC	short arm cast		
SACH	solid ankle cushion heel	SB-LM	Stanford Binet Intelligence Test-Form LM
SAD	sugar and acetone determination	SBO	small bowel obstruction
SAF	self-articulating femoral	SBP	systolic blood pressure; spontaneous bacterial peritonitis
Sag D	sagittal diameter		
SAH	subarachnoid hemorrhage; systemic arterial hypertension	SBR	strict bed rest
		SBT	serum bactericidal titers
SAL 12	sequential analysis of 12 chemistry constituents	SC	subcutaneous; subclavian; sickle-cell; Snellen's chart; subclavian; sternoclavicular; sulfur colloid; service connected
SAM	systolic anterior motion; self-administered medication		
		SCA	subcutaneous abdominal (block)
SAN	sinoatrial node		
sang	sanguinous	SCB	strictly confined to bed
SAPD	self-administration of psychotropic drugs	SCBC	small cell bronchogenic carcinoma
SAS	sulfasalazine; sleep apnea syndrome	SCC	squamous cell carcinoma; sickle cell crisis
SAT	saturation; Saturday; subacute thyroiditis	SCCa	squamous cell carcinoma
SAVD	spontaneous assisted vaginal delivery	SCCA	semi-closed circle absorber
SB	stillbirth; spina bifida; sternal border; stillborn; Sengstaken-Blakemore (tube); sinus bradycardia; small bowel	SCD	subacute combined degeneration; sickle cell disease; sudden cardiac death; service connected disability; spinal cord disease
		SCE	sister chromatid exchange
SBC	standard bicarbonate		
SBE	subacute bacterial endocarditis	SCG	sodium cromoglycate
		SCh	succinylcholine chloride
SBFT	small bowel follow through	SCI	spinal cord injury

SCID	severe combined immunodeficiency disorders	SE	side effect; Starr-Edwards
SCIV	subclavian intravenous	sec	secondary; secretary
SCLC	small-cell lung cancer	sed	sedimentation
		sed rt	sedimentation rate
SCLE	subcutaneous lupus erythematosis	SEER	Surveillance, Epidemiology, and End Results (program)
SCLs	soft contact lenses		
SCM	spondylitic caudal myelopathy; sterno-cleidomastoid	SEG	segment
		segs	segmented neutrophils
		SEM	systolic ejection murmur; scanning electron microscopy; standard error of mean
SCOP	scopolamine		
SCP	sodium cellulose phosphate		
		SEMI	subendocardial myocardial infarction
SCR	spondylitic caudal radiculopathy		
		SENS	sensorium
SCT	sickel cell trait; sugar coated tablet	SEP	separate; somato-sensory evoked potential; systolic ejection period
SCUT	schizophrenia chronic undifferentiated type		
		SER-IV	supination external rotation, type 4 fracture
SCV	subcutaneous vaginal (block)		
SD	standard deviation; spontaneous delivery; sterile dressing; scleroderma; surgical drain; senile dementia	SERs	somatosensory evoked responses
		SES	socioeconomic status
		SF	scarlet fever; sugar free; salt free; spinal fluid; symptom-free
S & D	stomach and duodenum		
SDA	Seventh-Day Adventist; steroid-dependent asthmatic	SFA	superficial femoral artery; saturated fatty acids
		SFC	spinal fluid count
SDAT	senile dementia of Alzheimer's type	SFEMG	single-fiber electro-myography
SDH	subdural hematoma	SFP	spinal fluid pressure
SDL	serum digoxin level	SFPT	standard fixation preference test
SDS	same day surgery		
SDT	Speech Detection Threshold	S.G.	specific gravity; Swan-Ganz; serum glucose

SGA	small for gestational age	SIJ	sacroiliac joint
SGD	straight gravity drainage	SIMV	synchronized intermittent mandatory ventilation
SGE	significant glandular enlargement	SIT	Slossen Intelligence Test; sperm immobilization test
s gl	without correction/ without glasses	SIW	self-inflicted wound
SGOT	serum glutamic oxaloacetic transaminase (same as AST)	SJS	Stevens-Johnson syndrome
		SK	streptokinase; SmithKline®
SGPT	serum glutamic pyruvic transaminase (same as ALT)	SK 65®	propoxyphene HCl 65 mg
SH	social history; serum hepatitis; shower; short; shoulder	SK-SD	streptokinase streptodornase
		SL	sublingual; slight
S&H	speech and hearing	SLB	short leg brace
S/H	suicidal/homicidal ideation	SLC	short leg cast
		SLE	systemic lupus erythematosus; slit lamp examination
SHA	super heated aerosol		
S Hb	sickle hemoglobin screen		
SHEENT	skin, head, eyes, ears, nose, throat	SLGXT	symptom limited graded exercise test
SHS	Student Health Service	SLK	superior limbic keratoconjunctivitis
SI	sacroiliac		
SIADH	syndrome of inappropriate antidiuretic hormone secretion	SLO	streptolysin O
		SLR	straight leg raising
		SLRT	straight leg raising test
S & I	suction and irrigation	SLWC	short leg walking cast
SIB	self-injurious behavior	SM	streptomycin; small; systolic murmur
sibs	siblings		
SICT	selective intracoronary thrombolysis	SMA	sequential multiple analyzer; simultaneous multichannel autoanalyzer; superior mesenteric artery; spinal muscular atrophy
SICU	surgical intensive care unit		
SIDS	sudden infant death syndrome		
Sig.	let it be marked (appears on prescription before directions for patient)		
		SMC	special mouth care
		SMD	senile macular degeneration

84

SMI	small volume infusion; sustained maximal inspiration	sol	solution
		SOM	serous otitis media
SMON	subacute myeloopticoneuropathy	SOMI	sterno-occipital mandibular immobilizer
		Sono	sonogram
SMP	self-management program	SONP	solid organs not palpable
SMR	submucosal resection; senior medical resident; standardized mortality ratio; skeletal muscle relaxant	SOP	standard operating procedure
		S.O.S.	may be repeated once if urgently required (Latin: si opus sit)
		SOT	stream of thought
SMS	senior medical student	SP	suprapubic; sequential pulse; sacrum to pubis
SMVT	sustained monomorphic ventricular tachycardia	
		S/P	status post
SN	student nurse	SPA	albumin human (formerly known as saltpoor albumin); stimulation produced analgesia
SNAP	sensory nerve action potential	
SNCV	sensory nerve conduction velocity	
		SPAG	small particle aerosol generator
SND	sinus node dysfunction	
SNE	subacute necrotizing encephalomyelopathy	SPBI	serum protein bound iodine
SNF	skilled nursing facility	SPBT	suprapubic bladder tap
SNGFR	single nephron glomerular filtration rate	SPE	serum protein electrolytes
SNP	sodium nitroprusside	SPEC	specimen
SNT	suppan nail technique	SPECT	single photon emission computer tomography
S-O	salpingo-oophorectomy	
SO₄	sulfate	Spec Ed	special education
SOA	swelling of ankles; supraorbital artery	SPEP	serum protein electrophoresis
SOAA	signed out against advice	SPF	sun protective factor
SOAP	subjective, objective, assessment and plans	sp fl	spinal fluid
		Sp.G.	specific gravity
SOB	shortness of breath	SPK	superficial punctate keratitis
S & OC	signed on and on chart (e.g. permit)	
SOD	superoxide dismutase; surgical officer of the day	SPMA	spinal progressive muscle atrophy

SPN	solitary pulmonary nodule	SRT	speech reception threshold; sedimentation rate test; sustained release theophylline
SPP	suprapubic prostatectomy		
SPROM	spontaneous premature rupture of membrane	SRU	side rails up
		SS	saline solution; sickle cell; half; social service; social security; salt substitute; slip sent; symmetrical strength
SPS	sodium polyethanol sulfanate		
SPT	skin prick test		
SP TAP	spinal tap		
SPU	short procedure unit		
SPVR	systemic peripheral vascular resistance		
SQ	subcutaneous (this is a dangerous abbreviation)	S&S	signs and symptoms; support & stimulation
		SSCA	single shoulder contrast arthrography
Sq CCa	squamous cell carcinoma	SSD	social security disability; source to skin distance; silver sulfadiazine
SR	sedimentation rate; sustained release; side rails; screen; system review; sinus rhythm		
		SSDI	social security disability income
SRBC	sheep red blood cells; sickle red blood cells	SSE	saline solution enema; soapsuds enema; systemic side effects
SRBOW	spontaneous rupture of bag of waters		
SRF	somatotropin releasing factor	SSEPs	somatosensory evoked potentials
		SSI	sub-shock insulin
SRF-A	slow releasing factor of anaphylaxis	SSKI	saturated solution potassium iodide
SRIF	somatotropin-release-inhibiting factor (Somatostatin)	SSM	superficial spreading melanoma
		SSOP	Second Surgical Opinion Program
SRMD	stress related mucosal damage	SSPE	subacute sclerosing panencephalitis
SR/NE	sinus rhythm, no ectopy	SSS	sick sinus syndrome; sterile saline soak
SROM	spontaneous rupture of membrane	SSSS	staphyloccal scalded skin syndrome
SRS-A	slow-reacting substance of anaphylaxis	SSX	sulfisoxazole acetyl

ST	speech therapist; sinus tachycardia; straight; split thickness	STS	serologic test for syphilis
STA	superficial temporal artery	STSG	split thickness skin graft
stab.	polymorphonuclear leukocytes (white blood cells) in nonmature form	STU	shock trauma unit
		STZ	streptozocin
		S&U	supine and upright
		SU	sensory urgency; Somogyi units
staph	Staphylococcus aureus	SUB	Skene's urethra and Bartholins glands
stat	immediately		
STB	stillborn	sub q	subcutaneous (this is a dangerous abbreviation since the q is mistaken for every, when a number follows)
ST BY	stand by		
STD	sexually transmitted diseases; skin test dose; sodium tetradecyl sulfate		
		SUD	sudden unexpected death
STD TF	standard tube feeding		
STET	submaximal treadmill exercise test	SUID	sudden unexplained infant death
STF	special tube feeding	SULF- PRIM	trimethoprim and sulfamethoxazole
STG	short-term goals		
STH	soft tissue hemorrhage; somatotrophic hormone	SUP	supinator; superior
		supp	suppository
STJ	subtalar joint	SUR	surgery, surgical
STM	short-term memory	SUX	succinylcholine
sTNM	surgical-evaluative staging of cancer	SV	single ventricle; stock volume; sigmoid volvulus
STNR	symmetrical tonic neck reflex		
		SVC	superior vena cava
STORCH	syphilis, toxoplasmosis, other agents, rubella, cytomegalovirus and herpes (maternal infections)	SVCO	superior vena cava obstruction
		SVD	spontaneous vaginal delivery
		SVE	sterile vaginal examination
STP	sodium thiopental		
STPD	standard temperature and pressure-dry	SVPB	supraventricular premature beat
strep	streptococcus; streptomycin	SVR	supraventricular rhythm; systemic vascular resistance

SVRI	systemic vascular resistance index		TAA	total ankle arthroplasty; triamcinolone acetonide; thoracic aortic aneurysm; tumor associated antigen (antibodies); transverse aortic arch
SVT	supraventricular tachycardia			
S.W.	social worker			
SWD	short wave diathermy			
SWFI	sterile water for injection			
SWI	sterile water for injection		TAB	tablet; triple antibiotic (bacitracin, neomycin and polymyxin- this is a dangerous abbreviation); therapeutic abortion
SWOG	Southwest Oncology Group			
SWS	student ward secretary; Sturge-Weber syndrome; slow wave sleep			
			TAC	triamicinolone cream
			TAD	transverse abdominal diameter
SWT	stab wound of the throat		TAE	transcatheter arterial embolization
Sx	signs; symptom; surgery		TAF	tissue angiogenesis factor
syr	syrup		TAH	total abdominal hysterectomy; total artificial heart
SZ	seizure; suction; schizophrenic			
SZN	streptozocin		TAL	tendon Achilles lengthening
			TAM	tamoxifen
			TANI	total axial (lymph) node irradiation

T

T	temperature		TAO	troleandomycin; thromboangitis obliterans
$T_{1/2}$	half-life			
T_1	tricuspid first sound; first thoracic vertebra			
T_3	triiodithyronine		TAPVC	total anomalous pulmonary venous connection
T_4	levothyroxine			
T-7	free thyroxine factor			
TA	therapeutic abortion; temperature axillary; tricuspid atresia		TAPVD	total anomalous pulmonary venous drainage
			TAPVR	total anomalous pulmonary venous return
Ta	tonometry applanation			
T&A	tonsillectomy and adenoidectomy		TAR	thrombocytopenia with absent radius
T(A)	axillary temperature			

TARA	total articular replacement arthroplasty
TAS	Therapeutic Activities Specialist
TAT	tetanus antitoxin; till all taken; Thematic Apperception Test
TB	tuberculosis
TBA	to be absorbed; to be admitted
TBB	transbronchial biopsy
tbc	tuberculosis
TBE	tick-born encephalitis
TBG	thyroxine-binding globulin
TBI	total body irradiation
T bili	total bilirubin
tbl.	tablespoon (15 mL)
TBM	tubule basement membrane
TBNA	treated but not admitted
TBPA	thyroxine-binding prealbumin
TBR	total bed rest
TBSA	total burn surface area
tbsp	tablespoon (15 mL)
TBV	total blood volume; transluminal balloon valvuloplasty
TBW	total body water
TBX_2	thromboxane B_2
TBX®	thiabendazole
T/C	to consider
TC	transcobalamin; true conjugate; tubocurarine; throat culture
Tc	technetium
T&C	type and crossmatch; turn and cough

TCA	tricyclic antidepressant; tricuspid atresia; terminal cancer; trichloroacetic acid
TCABG	triple coronary artery bypass graft
TCAD	tricyclic antidepressant
TCBS agar	thiosulfate-citrate-bile salt-sucrose agar
TCCB	transitional cell carcinoma of bladder
TCDB	turn, cough and deep breath
TCDD	tetrachlorodibenzo-p-dioxin
TCE	tetrachloroethylene
T cell	small lymphocyte
TCH	turn, cough, hyperventilate
TCID50	median tissue culture doses
TCM	transcutaneous monitor; tissue culture media
TCMH	tumor-direct cell-mediated hypersensitivity
TCMZ	trichloromethiazide
TCN	tetracycline
TCT	thyrocalcitonin
TCVA	thromboembolic cerebral vascular accident
TD	transverse diameter; tardive dyskinesia; tetanus-diphtheria toxoid (pediatric use); travelers diarrhea; treatment discontinued; tidal volume; Takayasu's disease
Td	tetanus-diphtheria toxoid (adult type)

TDD	thoracic duct drainage	TFT	trifluridine (trifluoro-thymidine)
TDE	total daily energy (requirement)	TFTs	thyroid function tests
TDF	tumor dose frac-tionation	TG	triglycerides
		6-TG	thioguanine
TDI	toluene diisocyanate	TGA	transient global am-nesia; transposition of the great arteries
TDK	tardive diskinesia		
TDM	therapeutic drug monitoring	TGFA	triglyceride fatty acid
TdP	torsade de pointes	TGS	tincture of green soap
TdR	Thymidine	TGT	thromboplastin genera-tion test
TDT	tentative discharge tomorrow		
		TH	thrill; total hysterec-tomy; thyroid hormone
TE	tracheoesophageal; trace elements		
		THA	total hip arthroplasty; transient hemispheric attack
T&E	trial and error		
TEA	total elbow arthro-plasty; thromboendar-terectomy		
		THAM®	tromethamine
		THC	transhepatic cholangio-gram; tetrahydro-cannibinol (dronabinol)
TEC	total eosinophil count		
TEDS®	Anti-embolism Stockings		
		TH-CULT	throat culture
TEF	tracheoesophageal fistula	THE	transhepatic embolization
TEG	thromboelastogram	Ther Ex	therapeutic exercise
tele	telemetry	THI	transient hypo-gammaglobinemia of infancy
TEM	transmission electron microscopy		
TEN	toxic epidermal necrolysis	THP	trihexphenidyl
		THR	total hip replacement
TEN®	Total Enteral Nutrition	TI	tricuspid insufficiency
TENS	transcutaneous electri-cal nerve stimulation	tib.	tibia
		TIA	transient ischemic attack
tert.	tertiary		
TES	Treatment Emergent Symptoms	TIBC	total iron-binding capacity
TESPA	thiotepa	tid	three times a day
TET	treadmill exercise test	TIE	transient ischemic episode
TF	tube feeding; to follow; tactile fremitus; tetral-ogy of Fallot		
		TIG	tetanus immune globulin
TFB	trifascicular block	tinct	tincture

+tive	positive	TNI	total nodal irradiation
TJ	triceps jerk	TNM	primary tumor, regional lymph nodes, distant metastasis (used with subscripts for the staging of cancer)
TJN	twin jet nebulizer		
TKA	total knee arthroplasty		
TKNO	to keep needle open		
TKP	thermokeratoplasty		
TKO	to keep open		
TKR	total knee replacement	TNTC	too numerous to count
TL	tubal ligation; team leader; trial leave		
		TO	telephone order
TLC	tender loving care; total lung capacity; total lymphocyte count; thin layer chromatography	T(O)	oral temperature
		TOA	tubo-ovarian abscess; time of arrival
		TOF	tetralogy of Fallot
		TOGV	transposition of the great vessels
TLI	total lymphoid irradiation	TOL	trial of labor
TLV	total lung volume	Tomo	tomography
TM	tympanic membrane; trabecular meshwork	TOP	termination of pregnancy
TMA	transmetatarsal amputation	TOPP	a drug combination protocol
TMB	transient monocular blindness	TOPV	trivalent oral polio vaccine
TMC	triamcinolone, Terramycin capsules; transmural colitis	TORCH	toxoplasmosis, other (syphillis, hepatitis, Zoster), rubella, cytomegalovirus, and herpes simplex (maternal infections)
TMET	tread mill exercise test		
TMI	threatened myocardial infarction		
TMJ	temporomandibular joint	TORP	total ossicular replacement prosthesis
TMP	trimethoprim; thallium myocardial perfusion	TOS	thoracic outlet syndrome
TMP/ SMX	trimethoprim-sulfamethoxazole	TP	total protein; Todd's paralysis
TMTC	too many to count	TPA	tissue plasminogen activator; total parenteral alimentation; tissue polypeptide antigen
TMX	tamoxifen		
Tn	normal intraocular tension		
TNF	tumor necrosis factor		
TNG	nitroglycerin	TPC	total patient care

TPD	tropical pancreatic diabetes	TRT	thermoradiotherapy
TPE	total protective environment	T3RU	triiodothyroxine resin uptake
TPH	thromboembolic pulmonary hypertension	TS	test solution; Tourette's syndrome
TPI	Treponema pallidium immobilization	TSA	total shoulder arthroplasty; toluenesulfonic acid
TPM	temporary pacemaker	TSAR®	tape surrounded Appli-rulers
TPN	total parenteral nutrition	TSBB	transtracheal selective bronchial brushing
TP & P	time, place and person		
TPPN	total peripheral parenteral nutrition	TSD	Tay-Sachs disease; target to skin distance
TPR	temperature, pulse, and respiration; temperature; total peripheral resistance	T set	tracheotomy set
		TSF	tricep skin fold
		TSH	thyroid-stimulating hormone
TPT	time to peak tension	tsp	teaspoon (5 ml)
TPVR	total peripheral vascular resistance	TSP	total serum protein
		TSPA	thiotepa
Tr	trace; tincture; tremor; treatment	TSR	total shoulder replacement
T(R)	rectal temperature	TSS	toxic shock syndrome
TRA	therapeutic recreation associate	TST	titmus stereocuity test
		T&T	touch and tone
trach.	tracheal; tracheostomy	TT	transtracheal; thrombin time; tetanus toxoid; tilt table; twitch tension; thymol turbidity
Trans D	transverse diameter		
TRC	tanned red cells		
TRD	traction retinal detachment		
Tren	Trendelenberg	T/T	trace of __/trace of __
TRH	thyrotropin-releasing hormone	TT4	total thyroxine
		TTA	total toe arthroplasty
TRIG	triglycerides	TTN	transient tachypnea of the newborn
TRM- SMX	trimethoprim– sulfamethoxazole	TTNB	transient tachypnea of the newborn
tRNA	transfer ribonucleic acid	TTP	thrombotic thrombocytopenic purpura
TRP	tubular reabsorption of phosphate	TTS	through the skin

TTVP	temporary transvenous pacemaker
TU	tuberculin units
TUR	transurethral resection
T$_3$UR	triiodothyronine uptake ratio
TURB	turbidity
TURBN	transurethral resection bladder neck
TURBT	transurethral resection bladder tumor
TURP	transurethral resection of prostate
TURV	transurethral resection valves
TV	trial visit; Trichomonas vaginalis; tidal volume
TVC	triple voiding cystogram; true vocal cord
TVH	total vaginal hysterectomy
TVP	transvenous pacemaker
TW	test weight
TWD	total white and differential count
TWE	tapwater enema
TWETC	tapwater enema till clear
TWWD	tap water wet dressing
Tx	treatment; therapy; traction; transfuse; transplant
TxA$_2$	thromboxane A$_2$
Tyl	tyloma (callus); Tylenol®
TYCO #3	Tylenol® with 30 mg of codeine (#1=7.5 mg, #2=15 mg and #4=60 mg of codeine present

U

U	units (this is the most dangerous abbreviation—spell out "unit"); ultralente insulin; urine
U/1	1 finger breadth below umbilicus
1/U	1 finger over umbilicus
U/	at umbilicus
UA	uric acid; urinalysis; unauthorized absence; uncertain about
UAC	umbilical artery catheter
UAL	umbilical artery line
UAO	upper airway obstruction
UAT	up as tolerated
UAVC	univentricular atrioventricular connection
UBF	unknown black female
UBI	ultraviolet blood irradiation
UBM	unknown black male
UC	urine culture; uterine contraction; ulcerative colitis
U&C	urethral & cervical
UCD	usual childhood diseases
UCG	urinary chorionicgonadotropins
UCHD	usual childhood diseases
UCI	urethral catheter in
UCO	urethral catheter out
UCX	urine culture
UD	urethral discharge

UDC	usual diseases of childhood	urol	urology
UE	upper extremity	US	ultrasonography; unit secretary
UES	upper esophageal sphincter	USA	United States Army; unit services assistant
UFO	unflagged order	USAF	United States Air Force
UG	urogenital	USB	upper sternal border
UGDP	University Group Diabetes Project	USG	ultrasonography
UGH	uveitis, glaucoma, hyphema	USI	urinary stress incontinence
UGI	upper gastrointestinal series	USMC	United States Marine Corp
UHBI	upper hemibody irradiation	USN	ultrasonic nebulizer; United States Navy
UHDDS	Uniform Hospital Discharge Data Set	USP	United States Pharmacopeia
UID	once daily (this is a dangerous abbreviation, spell out "once daily")	UTD	up to date
		ut dict	as directed
		UTF	usual throat flora
		UTI	urinary tract infection
UIQ	upper inner quadrant	UTO	upper tibial osteotomy
U/L	upper and lower	UTZ	ultrasound
U & L	upper and lower	UUN	urine urea nitrogen
ULN	upper limits of normal	UV	ultraviolet
ULQ	upper left quadrant	UVA	ureterovesical angle; ultraviolet A light
UK	unknown; urokinase	UVB	ultraviolet B light
umb ven	umbilical vein	UVC	umbilical vein catheter
UN	urinary nitrogen	UVJ	ureterovesical junction
UNA	urinary nitrogen appearance; urine sodium	UVL	ultraviolet light
		UWF	unknown white female
ung	ointment	UWM	unknown white male
UNK	unknown		
UOQ	upper outer quadrant		
UPJ	ureteropelvic junction		

V

V	vomiting; vein; five; vagina
U/P ratio	urine to plasma ratio		
UPT	urine pregnancy test		
UR	utilization review	VA	visual acuity; Veterans Administration; valproic acid; vacuum aspiration
URI	upper respiratory infection		
url	unrelated		

VAC	vincristine, Adriamycin®, cyclophosphamide; ventriculo-arterial connections	VCUG	vesicoureterogram; voiding cysto-urethrogram
VAD	vascular (venous) access device	VD	venereal disease; volume of distribution; voided
vag.	vagina	VDA	visual discriminatory acuity; venous digital angiogram
VAG HYST	vaginal hysterectomy	VDG	venereal disease—gonorrhea
VAH	Veterans Administration Hospital	Vdg	voiding
VAMC	Veterans Administration Medical Center	VDH	valvular disease of the heart
VAPA	a drug combination protocol	VDRL	Venereal Disease Research Laboratory (test for syphilis)
VAR	variant	VDRR	vitamin D-resistant rickets
VAS	vascular; visual analogue scale	VDS	vindesine; venereal disease—syphilis
VASC	Visual-Auditory Screen Test for Children	VDT	video display terminal
VAS RAD	vascular radiology	VE	vaginal examination; vertex
VB	Van Buren (catheter)	VEB	ventricular ectopic beat
VBAC	vaginal birth after cesarean	VEE	Venezuelan equine encephalitis
VBD	vinblastine, bleomycin and cisplatin	vent.	ventricular; ventral
VBI	vertebrobasilar insufficiency	VEP	visual evoked potential
VBL	vinblastine	VER	visual evoked responses; ventricular escape rhythm
VBS	vertebral-basilar system	VF	vision field; ventricular fibrillation; vocal fremitus
VC	vital capacity; vena cava; vocal cords; color vision	V. Fib	ventricular fibrillation
VCG	vectocardiography	VFP	vitreous fluoro-photometry
VCR	vincristine sulfate	VG	vein graft; very good; ventricular gallop
VCT	venous clotting time		
VCU	voiding cystourethrogram		

VH	vaginal hysterectomy; viral hepatitis; Veterans Hospital; vitreous hemorrhage	VP	venous pressure; variegate porphyria; ventriculoperitoneal; ventricular-peritoneal
VI	volume index; six	V & P	ventilation and perfusion; vagotomy and pyloroplasty
vib	vibration		
VID	videodensitometry	VP-16	etoposide
VIG	vaccinia immune globulin	VPA	valproic acid
		VPB	ventricular premature beat
VIP	voluntary interruption of pregnancy; vasoactive intestinal peptide	VPC	ventricular premature contractions
		VPDs	ventricular premature depolarizations
VISC	vitreous infusion suction cutter	VPL	vento-posterolateral
VIT	vitamin; vital; venom immunotherapy	VR	verbal reprimand; ventricular rhythm
vit. cap.	vital capacity	VS	vital signs; versus
VKC	vernal keratoconjunctivitis	VSD	ventricular septal defect
VLBW	very low birth weight	VSR	venous stasis retinopathy
VLDL	very low density lipoprotein	VSS	vital signs stable
VLH	ventrolateral nucleus of the hypothalamus	VT	ventricular tachycardia
		v. tach.	ventricular tachycardia
VM 26	teniposide	VTE	venous thromboembolism
VMA	vanillylmandelic acid		
VMH	ventromedial hypothalamus	VTX	vertex
		VV	varicose veins
VNA	Visiting Nurses' Association	V&V	vulva and vagina
VO	verbal order	V/V	volume to volume ratio
VOCTOR	void on call to operating room	VVFR	vesicovaginal fistula repair
VOD	vision right eye; venocclusive disease	VVOR	visual-vestibulo-ocular-reflex
VOL	voluntary	VW	vessel wall
VOR	vestibular ocular reflex	VWM	ventricular wall motion
VOS	vision left eye	VZ	varicella zoster
VOU	vision both eyes		

| VZIG | varicella zoster immune globulin |
| VZV | varicella zoster virus |

W

w	white; widowed; with
WA	while awake; when awake
WAIS	Wechsler Adult Intelligence Scale
WAIS-R	Wechsler Adult Intelligence Scale-Revised
WAP	wandering atrial pacemaker
WAS	Wishott-Aldrich syndrome
WASS	Wasserman test
WB	whole blood; weight bearing
WBAT	weight bearing as tolerated
WBC	white blood cell (count)
WBH	whole-body hyperthermia
WBN	wellborn nursery
WC	wheelchair; white count; ward clerk; whooping cough
W/D	warm and dry; withdrawal
W→D	wet to dry
WDHA	watery diarrhea, hypokalemia, and achlorhydria
WDLL	well-differentiated lymphocytic lymphoma
WDWN-BM	well-developed, well-nourished black male

WDWN-WF	well-developed, well-nourished white female
WE	weekend
WEE	western equine encephalitis
WEP	weekend pass
WF	white female
WFI	water for injection
WFL	within functional limits
WFR	wheel-and-flare reaction
WHO	World Health Organization
WHV	woodchuck hepatitis virus
WHVP	wedged hepatic venous pressure
WIA	wounded in action
WIC	women, infants and children
WID	widow; widower
WISC	Welcher Intelligence Scale for Children
WLS	wet lung syndrome
WLT	waterload test
WK	week
WKS	Wernicke-Korsakoff syndrome
WM	white male
WMA	wall motion abnormality
WN	well nourished
WND	wound
WNL	within normal limits
W/O	without
WO	written order; weeks old
W.P.	whirlpool
WPFM	Wright peak flow meter
WPP	Welcher Preschool Primary Scale of Intelligence

WPW	Wolff-Parkinson-White
WR	Wasserman reaction; wrist
WS	ward secretary; watt seconds
wt.	weight
WWAC	walk with aid of cane
W/U	workup
W/V	weight-to-volume ratio
W/W	weight-to-weight ratio

X

X	times; ten; start of anesthesia; crossmatch; break; except
X3	orientation as to time, place and person
X&D	examination and diagnosis
XM	crossmatch
X-mat.	crossmatch (blood)
XMM	xeromammorgraphy
XRT	radiotherapy
XS-LIM	exceeds limits of procedure
XT	exotropia
XV	fifteen
XX	twenty; normal female sex chromosome type
XXX	thirty
XY	normal male sex chromosome type

Y

YACP	young adult chronic patient
YAG	yittrium aluminum garnert (laser)
YF	yellow fever
YJV	yellow jacket venom
YLC	youngest living child
YO	years old
YORA	younger-onset rheumatoid arthritis
YSC	yolk sac carcinoma

Z

Z-E	Zollinger-Ellison
ZEEP	zero end-expiratory pressure
ZES	Zellinger-Ellison syndrome
Z-ESR	zeta erythrocyte sedimentation rate
ZIG	zoster serum immune globulin
ZIP	zoster immune plasma
ZMC	zygomatic
Zn	zinc
ZnO	zinc oxide
ZnOE	zinc oxide & eugenol
ZPC	zopiclone

Miscellaneous

↑	increase; alive; high; above; elevated; greater than; rising
↓	decrease; dead; restricted; normal plantar reflex; falling
→	results in; to the right; progressing to; showed
←	to the left
⟷	unchanging; stable
↓↓	testes descended; flexor
↑↑	extensor; testes undescended
||	parallel
#	number; fracture; pound
∴	therefore
Δ scan	delta scan (CT scan)
+	plus; positive
−	minus; negative
±	plus or minus; either positive or negative; very slight trace
>	greater than
≥	greater than or equal to
<	less than
≤	less than or equal to
≮	not less than
≯	not more than
∧	diastolic blood pressure; approximately
∨	systolic blood pressure
≠	not equal to

≅	approximately equal to
≈	approximately
?	questionable
∅	none; no
@	at
1°	primary; first degree
2°	secondary; second degree
3°	tertiary; third degree
i	one
ii	two
iii	three
iv	four
v	five
vi	six
vii	seven
viii	eight
ix	nine
x	ten
xi	eleven
xii	twelve
♂	male
♀	female
◇	sex unknown
□	male (father, brother, son)
○	female (mother, sister, daughter); respirations
(□)	adopted
*	birth
†	death; dead
⚲	standing
○—<	recumbent position
	sitting position
Α α	alpha
Β β	beta
Γ γ	gamma

Δ δ	delta; change; anion gap; delta gap; temperature	$\dfrac{140 \mid 101 \mid 17}{3.4 \mid 25 \mid 140}$	Na = 140, Cl = 101, BUN = 17 K = 3.4, CO₂ = 25, glucose = 140 (the positions can vary)
E ε	epsilon		
Z ζ	zeta		
H η	eta	$5.0 \diagup{\overset{16 \mid 85}{45 \mid 30}}\diagdown 35$	red blood cell count, hemoglobin, mean corpuscular volume, mean corpuscular hemoglobin concentration, hematocrit, mean corpuscular hemoglobin
Θ θ	theta		
I ι	iota		
K κ	kappa		
Λ λ	lambda		
M μ	mu; micro		
N ν	nu		
Ξ ξ	xi		
O o	omicron		
Π π	pi	$\dfrac{2\ cm \mid 80\%}{-2\ Vtx}$	2 cm = dilation of cervix
P ρ	rho		
Σ σ ς	sigma; sum of		80% = degree of cervix effacement
T τ	tau		
Υ υ	upsilon		Vtx = vertex; presentation of fetus, (breech = Br)
Φ φ	phi; phenyl		
X χ	chi		
Ψ ψ	psi; psychiatric		−2 = station; distance above (−) or below (+) the spine of the ischium measured in cm
Ω ω	omega		
′	feet; minutes (as in 30′)		
″	inches; seconds		
⊙	start of an operation		
⊗	end of anesthesia		

Reflexes[4]

Reflexes are usually graded on a 0 to 4+ scale:

4+	very brisk, hyperactive; may indicate disease; often associated with clonus
3+	brisker than average; possibly but not necessarily indicative of disease
2+	average; normal
1+	somewhat diminished; low normal
0	no response; may indicate neuropathy

Pulse[4]

0	completely absent
+1	markedly impaired
+2	moderately impaired
+3	slightly impaired
+4	normal

Gradation of intensity of heart murmurs[4]

1/6 or I/VI	very faint, heard only after the listener has "tuned in"; may not be heard in all positions
2/6 or II/VI	quiet but heard immediately upon placing the stethoscope on the chest
3/6 or III/VI	moderately loud
4/6 or IV/VI	loud
5/6 or V/VI	very loud, may be heard with a stethoscope partly off the chest (thrills are associated)
6/6 or VI/VI	may be heard with the stethoscope entirely off the chest (thrills are associated)

Apothecary symbols

The symbols presented below are for informational use. The apothecary system should *not* be used. Only the metric system should be used. The methods of expressing the symbols, the meanings, and the equivalences are not the classic ones, nor are they accurate, but reflect the usual intended meanings when used by some older physicians in writing prescription directions.

ℨ or ℨ ｉ	dram, teaspoonful, 5 ml	℥ or ℥ ｉ	ounce, 30 ml
		gr	grain (approximately 60 mg)
ℨ ｉｉ	two drams, 2 teaspoonfuls, 10 ml	ℳ	minim (approximately 0.06 ml)
℥ ss	half ounce, tablespoonful, 15 ml	gtt	drop

101

Please forward any additional meanings for these abbreviations, additional abbreviations and their meanings, or corrections to the author so that the list can be updated. Thank you. Dr. Neil M. Davis, 1143 Wright Drive, Huntingdon Valley, PA 19006.

PRICE

1-4 copies	$5.95 each	(check or money order must accompany order)
5-14 copies	$5.95 each	(Purchase order accepted)
20 or more copies	$4.25 each	(Purchase order accepted)

United States—Postage and handling charges are included. Pennsylvania residents add 6% sales tax.
Outside the United States—Prices as shown above plus postage. Pay in U.S. dollars through a correspondent U.S. bank.

Order from
Neil M. Davis Associates
1143 Wright Drive
Huntingdon Valley, PA 19006
Phone (215) 947-1862 or 1752